AF514599

Biomarkers of Cardiometabolic Risk, Inflammation and Disease

Filipe Palavra • Flávio Reis • Daniela Marado
Armando Sena
Editors

Biomarkers of Cardiometabolic Risk, Inflammation and Disease

Springer

Editors
Filipe Palavra
Laboratory of Pharmacology and Experimental Therapeutics
Institute for Biomedical Imaging and Life Sciences (IBILI) and CNC.IBILI Research Unit
Faculty of Medicine, Coimbra University
Coimbra, Portugal

Flávio Reis
Laboratory of Pharmacology and Experimental Therapeutics
Institute for Biomedical Imaging and Life Sciences (IBILI) and CNC.IBILI Research Unit
Faculty of Medicine, Coimbra University
Coimbra, Portugal

Daniela Marado
Department of Internal Medicine – B
Centro Hospitalar e Universitário de Coimbra
Coimbra, Portugal

Armando Sena
Interdisciplinary Centre of Research Egas Moniz, CiiEM
Caparica, Portugal

ISBN 978-3-319-16017-7 ISBN 978-3-319-16018-4 (eBook)
DOI 10.1007/978-3-319-16018-4

Library of Congress Control Number: 2015937599

Springer Cham Heidelberg New York Dordrecht London
© Springer International Publishing Switzerland 2015
This work is subject to copyright. All rights are reserved by the Publisher, whether the whole or part of the material is concerned, specifically the rights of translation, reprinting, reuse of illustrations, recitation, broadcasting, reproduction on microfilms or in any other physical way, and transmission or information storage and retrieval, electronic adaptation, computer software, or by similar or dissimilar methodology now known or hereafter developed.
The use of general descriptive names, registered names, trademarks, service marks, etc. in this publication does not imply, even in the absence of a specific statement, that such names are exempt from the relevant protective laws and regulations and therefore free for general use.
The publisher, the authors and the editors are safe to assume that the advice and information in this book are believed to be true and accurate at the date of publication. Neither the publisher nor the authors or the editors give a warranty, express or implied, with respect to the material contained herein or for any errors or omissions that may have been made.

Printed on acid-free paper

Springer International Publishing AG Switzerland is part of Springer Science+Business Media (www.springer.com)

Preface

Cardiovascular diseases are among the leading causes of permanent disability and death worldwide. In recent years, an extraordinary effort has been made, in terms of public health, to optimize the prevention of these diseases and to minimize the major risk factors that are associated with them. We have never been so aggressive in fighting against sedentary lifestyle, obesity, smoking, arterial hypertension and metabolic dysregulation (especially considering diabetes mellitus and dyslipidemia). However, the impact of such measures on the epidemiology (particularly on the incidence) of these diseases has not been as strong as desired. They continue to be responsible for high costs worldwide, not only from a personal viewpoint but also from family and social perspectives.

For all this, the scientific community has invested a lot in the study of these diseases, particularly of the risk factors that are associated with them, and clinicians have been provided with increasingly interesting tools for effective cardiometabolic risk stratification. Knowledge in this area has advanced at an extraordinary pace, and today there are new molecules and new markers that may help to further refine the whole process of risk stratification (cytokines and C-reactive protein levels, for example). Additionally, many of these markers are related to chronic inflammation, and the impact they have on cardiovascular diseases is spreading to the study of diseases typically characterized by a state of chronic inflammation. Implications of this knowledge are transversal to all areas of medicine that directly deal with these clinical entities – from neurology to cardiology, considering also internal medicine, rheumatology, and nephrology, all clinicians have to update themselves with this information and to rapidly incorporate these concepts into practice.

With this book, we intend to present, in an organized and systematic way, all the advances that have been achieved in this area over the past few years. It starts with a chapter covering some relevant concepts that help to understand the relationship between chronic inflammation and cardiometabolic risk; then it goes through cardiovascular diseases (with a special focus on atherosclerosis and atrial fibrillation), type 2 diabetes mellitus and metabolic syndrome, ischemic stroke, chronic kidney disease, and systemic autoimmune disorders; and it ends with a chapter devoted to very recent aspects merging chronic inflammation, cardiometabolic risk, and neurodegenerative diseases. With this work, we believe we are creating an important study tool for all clinicians who, in practice, need to deal with these diseases. Transversality is one of its features, because various medical specialties are in need for this knowledge to be compiled into a single work, presenting it in an organized and easy-to-read way.

Coimbra, Portugal Filipe Palavra
Coimbra, Portugal Flávio Reis
Coimbra, Portugal Daniela Marado
Caparica, Portugal Armando Sena

Contents

Editors and Contributors

Editors and Contributors

Filipe Palavra, M.D. Laboratory of Pharmacology and Experimental Therapeutics, Institute for Biomedical Imaging and Life Sciences (IBILI) and CNC.IBILI Research Unit, Faculty of Medicine, Sub-Unit 1 (Pólo III), Coimbra University, Coimbra, Portugal

Flávio Reis, Ph.D. Laboratory of Pharmacology and Experimental Therapeutics, Institute for Biomedical Imaging and Life Sciences (IBILI) and CNC.IBILI Research Unit, Faculty of Medicine, Sub-Unit 1 (Pólo III), Coimbra University, Coimbra, Portugal

Daniela Marado, M.D. Department of Internal Medicine – B, Centro Hospitalar e Universitário de Coimbra, Coimbra, Portugal

Armando Sena, M.D., Ph.D. Interdisciplinary Centre of Research Egas Moniz, CiiEM, Caparica, Portugal

Contributors

Rui Alves, M.D., Ph.D. Universitary Nephrology Unit, Faculty of Medicine, University of Coimbra, Coimbra, Portugal

Adam J. Chicco, Ph.D. Department of Health and Exercise and Biomedical Sciences, Colorado State University, Fort Collins, CO, USA

Ana Cristina Cordeiro, M.D. Department of Rheumatology, Hospital Garcia de Orta, Almada, Portugal

Elísio Costa, Ph.D. UCIBIO, REQUIMTE, Laboratory of Biochemistry, Department of Biological Sciences, Faculty of Pharmacy, University of Porto, Porto, Portugal

Diana Aguiar de Sousa, M.D., M.Sc. Department of Neurology, Hospital de Santa Maria, University of Lisbon, Lisbon, Portugal

Ethel Ciampi Díaz, M.D. Department of Neurology, Hospital Clinico Pontificia Universidad Catolica de Chile, Santiago, Chile

Andreia Fernandes, M.D. Department of Cardiology – B, Centro Hospitalar e Universitário de Coimbra, Coimbra, Portugal

José M. Ferro, M.D., Ph.D. Department of Neurology, Hospital de Santa Maria, University of Lisbon, Lisbon, Portugal

Ana Catarina Fonseca, M.D., Ph.D., M.P.H. Department of Neurology, Hospital de Santa Maria, University of Lisbon, Lisbon, Portugal

Pablo M. Garcia-Roves, Ph.D. Department of Physiological Sciences II, Faculty of Medicine, University of Barcelona, L'Hospitalet Llobregat, Spain

Victor M. Gil, M.D., Ph.D. Department of Cardiology, Hospital dos Lusíadas, Lisbon, Portugal

Lino Gonçalves, M.D., Ph.D. Department of Cardiology – B, Centro Hospitalar e Universitário de Coimbra, Coimbra, Portugal

Alba Gonzalez-Franquesa, M.Sc., Ph.D. Diabetes and Obesity Laboratory, Institut d'Investigacions Biomèdiques August Pi I Sunyer (IDIBAPS), Barcelona, Spain

Leticia Martín-Cordero, Ph.D. Department of Nursing (Immunophysiology Research Group), University of Extremadura, Badajoz, Spain

Eduardo Ortega, Ph.D. Department of Physiology (Immunophysiology Research Group), Faculty of Sciences, University of Extremadura, Badajoz, Spain

Rui Providência, M.D., M.Sc. Department of Cardiology – B, Centro Hospitalar e Universitário de Coimbra, Coimbra, Portugal

Maria José Santos, M.D., Ph.D. Department of Rheumatology, Hospital Garcia de Orta, Almada, Portugal

Alice Santos-Silva, Ph.D. UCIBIO, REQUIMTE, Laboratory of Biochemistry, Department of Biological Sciences, Faculty of Pharmacy, University of Porto, Porto, Portugal

Chapter 1
Inflammation Biomarkers and Cardiometabolic Risk

Flávio Reis and Filipe Palavra

Abstract The ominous presence of inflammation in all phases of atherosclerosis has prompted the evaluation of emergent biomarkers of inflammation as tools to help in identifying patients at high risk for future cardiovascular events, to improve diagnostic and prognostic abilities, and to monitor disease activity and efficacy of therapy. Acute-phase reactants, pro- and anti-inflammatory cytokines, cell adhesion molecules, chemokines, and other mediators involved in the pathogenesis of atherosclerosis have been shown to have predictive value to determine future cardiovascular events and/or death, but until now, none, with the exception of hsCRP, has demonstrated additive value to the Framingham Risk Score.

Keywords Inflammation • Atherosclerosis • Cardiometabolic risk • Biomarkers

Inflammation in Health and Disease: Overview

Inflammation, derived from the Latin word *inflammare*, means "to set on fire." Inflammation is a part of the host defense system that counteracts insults incurred by internal or external stimuli, and the typical clinical signs include redness, heat, swelling, pain, and loss of function. Inflammation is not injurious in its essence and is necessary for the removal of challenges faced by the organism and consequent homeostasis restoration. In fact, the inflammatory responsiveness should be viewed as part of the physiological mechanisms operating to respond to stress experienced by cells, tissues, and organs.

Inflammation can be classified as acute or chronic. Chronic and acute inflammatory processes were traditionally thought to be motivated by different causes, through the activities of different cells and mediators, resulting in different outcomes. Nevertheless, a more modern vision indicates that processes are connected

F. Reis, Ph.D. (✉) • F. Palavra, M.D.
Laboratory of Pharmacology and Experimental Therapeutics, Institute for Biomedical Imaging and Life Sciences (IBILI) and CNC.IBILI Research Unit, Faculty of Medicine, Sub-Unit 1 (Pólo III), University of Coimbra, Coimbra 3000-548, Portugal
e-mail: freis@fmed.uc.pt

© Springer International Publishing Switzerland 2015

F. Palavra et al. (eds.), *Biomarkers of Cardiometabolic Risk, Inflammation and Disease*, DOI 10.1007/978-3-319-16018-4_1

in order to give organisms the ability to deal with distinct insults in a robust and flexible manner, thus regulating key homeostatic functions [1].

Acute inflammation is an immediate response of the body and is required to remove injurious pathogens. Facing infection, tissue damage, or acute inflammation, the host undergoes a series of biochemical and physiological changes known as acute-phase response. This process involves a cascade of events and is mediated by several distinct cells and molecules that locate pathogens or damaged tissue, recruit other cells and molecules, and then eliminate harmful agents, finally restoring body equilibrium. In brief, in a normal inflammatory response, tissue injury induces the release into the surrounding area of pro-inflammatory mediators, such as tumor necrosis factor (TNF)-α, interleukin (IL)-1β, IL-6, histamine, leukotrienes, and prostaglandins, by mast cells and resident macrophages, resulting in vasodilation and leaky blood vessels. Complement plasma proteins are released and call for phagocytic cells (i.e., monocytes and neutrophils) to the area to remove necrotic tissue, invading bacteria, and debris. The final step of inflammation is resolution and occurs due to neutrophil-evoked conversion of prostaglandins and leukotrienes in lipoxins, thus initiating the termination sequence, as well as due to production and release of anti-inflammatory factors, such as transforming growth factor (TGF)-β and IL-10, by activated macrophages. In addition, neutrophils and reparative fibroblasts infiltrate the area, releasing matrix metalloproteinases (MMPs) for tissue remodeling and producing extracellular matrix (ECM) and collagen. Macrophages finally leave the site through lymph vessels. When these steps are firmly followed, acute inflammation resolves without tissue damage [2].

When inflammation persists for a longer time, the type of cells at the site of damage changes, leading to chronic inflammation, which is a delayed response. Chronic inflammation involves persistent acute inflammation due to a deregulated resolution phase, which could result from incapacity to remove the inflammatory stimulus, an incessant procession of leukocytes which are responsible for the production of pro-inflammatory cytokines and reactive oxygen species (ROS) that persistently damage and remodel tissue, as well as due to a condition that maintains leukocytes at the site of inflammation [2].

Chronic inflammatory diseases (which are known to initiate due to persistent or deregulated inflammation) define an extremely important part of human pathology, and several examples can be cited as follows: asthma, systemic lupus erythematosus, rheumatoid arthritis, prostatitis, ulcerative colitis, Crohn's disease, wound healing, reperfusion injury, sarcoidosis, transplant rejection, vasculitis, chronic obstructive pulmonary disease, psoriasis, sepsis, cancer, Alzheimer's disease, as well as atherosclerosis, diabetes, and obesity [2].

Numerous molecules and factors are implicated in the regulation of inflammation at the molecular level, including cytokines (such as IL-l, IL-2, IL-6, IL-12, and TNF-α), chemokines (i.e., monocyte chemoattractant protein 1, IL-8), pro-inflammatory transcription factors (NF-κB, STAT3) and enzymes (COX-2, 5-LOX, 12-LOX, MMPs), prostate-specific antigen (PSA), C-reactive protein, adhesion molecules (intercellular adhesion molecule-1 [ICAM-l], vascular cell adhesion molecule-1 [VCAM-1], endothelial leukocyte adhesion molecule [ELAM-1]), vascular endothelial growth factor (VEGF), and TWIST. During the last year, several of these mediators and factors have been studied as putative disease/risk markers in distinct inflammatory conditions, including in cardiovascular and metabolic disorders.

Inflammation and Cardiometabolic Risk

Regardless of the availability of successful treatment strategies for dyslipidemia and hypertension, cardiovascular diseases (CVD) account for one-third of all deaths worldwide, and prevalence still increases [3]. CVD comprise a class of diseases that involve heart and systemic blood vessels. In coronary heart disease, cerebrovascular disease, or peripheral arterial disease, impaired blood vessel function leads to an inadequate blood supply of organs. Several factors influence the risk of developing CVD, including lifestyle habits (such as unhealthy diet, physical inactivity, smoking, obesity, diabetes, high blood pressure, and dyslipidemia) as well as genetic, epigenetic, and environmental factors.

Atherosclerosis is the most common pathological process that leads to CVD, including myocardial infarction (MI), heart failure, stroke, and claudication. A central event is the development of atherosclerotic plaques in the inner lining of arteries, which is characterized by necrotic cores, calcification, and accumulation of modified lipids and foam cells, but also other cell types such as smooth muscle cells, vascular dendritic cells, T cells, and endothelial cells are involved in lesion formation [4]. The multifactorial background makes it difficult to unravel initial pathological events, which are suggested to occur in a variety of cell types in a very early phase of disease, when symptoms are subclinical. While in the past atherosclerosis was viewed primarily as a passive process of cholesterol accumulation, recent evidence indicates that it is a highly active process involving components of the vascular, immune, metabolic, and endocrine systems [4].

Even though the conventional risk factors (age, male sex, hypercholesterolemia, hypertension, and smoking) in the Framingham Risk Score (FRS) account for most of the risk of coronary heart disease (CHD), about one-third of individuals with none or only one risk factor indeed develop CHD, and up to 40 % of subjects with cholesterol levels below the population average die from CHD [5, 6]. In addition, many cardiovascular (CV) events occur in patients treated with statin therapy [7]. Regardless the important role of cholesterol in atherosclerosis, many individuals who experience acute MI present total and/or LDL cholesterol below thresholds. Statin therapy alone appears to be insufficient in decreasing the high level of residual risk of further CV events, which remains at 50–75 % of that of control groups [7]. In addition, absolute CV risk remains high: about one in six patients treated with a statin in monotherapy experiences further events over a 5-year period [7], and one in five patients with a history of acute coronary syndrome who is treated with a statin dies within 30 months [8]. This convergence of clinical findings highlights the need for improving our ability to predict CV risk.

A major shift in the paradigm of our understanding of the pathogenesis of atherosclerosis has been seen in the last decade. The biology of the atherosclerotic plaque, rather than the degree of stenosis, is now recognized as a pivotal feature in determining plaque stability. Inflammatory mechanisms play a crucial role in all phases of atherosclerosis, from initial recruitment of circulating leucocytes to the arterial wall to eventual rupture of the unstable plaque. An abundant presence of inflammatory cells, including monocyte-derived macrophages and T lymphocytes, was found at the site of rupture or superficial erosion, which is preceded by endothelial cell dysfunction with production of adhesion molecules that interact with inflammatory cells [9, 10]. Macrophages secrete various cytokines, chemokines, growth factors, and disintegrins that cause activation and proliferation of smooth muscle cells (SMCs) and lesion progression; finally, weakening of vulnerable plaque occurs by matrix degradation of its fibrous cap [11]. Several factors are found in the atherosclerotic plaque maintaining and amplifying the inflammatory mechanisms in the atherosclerotic region, including adipocytokines, angiotensin II (ANG II), heat shock proteins (HSPs), immune complexes, ROS, and pro-inflammatory cytokines.

Advances in vascular biology have established the interaction of the innate immune system with atherosclerosis; in fact, inflammation is pivotal to the initiation and progression of atherothrombosis and to triggering CVD [12–14]. Inflammation in cells involved in atherosclerosis is elicited by many other risk factors associated with atherosclerosis, including cigarette smoking, insulin resistance/diabetes, and arterial hypertension [15]. Thus, the inflammatory pathways involved in both innate and adaptive immune responses appear to transduce many of the traditional risk factors for atherosclerosis.

The ominous presence of inflammation in atherosclerosis has prompted the evaluation of emergent biomarkers of inflammation as tools to help in identifying patients at high risk for future CV events.

Epidemiologic, experimental, preclinical, and clinical studies have led to the identification of key non-modifiable and modifiable risk factors for CVD, which were able to allow discrimination of risk between individuals and serve as basis for scores of risk calculators, being the most widely used the FRS. However, the burden of obesity and diabetes has been changing the way we classically look for CV risk factors. Organizations around the world have defined the metabolic syndrome (MetS) as a cluster of metabolic abnormalities, with insulin resistance and adiposity as central features [16, 17]. Diagnostic criteria for MetS have been defined by the National Cholesterol Education Program Adult Treatment Panel III (NCEP-ATP III): central obesity, dyslipidemia (high triglycerides, low high-density lipoprotein [HDL] cholesterol), hypertension, and impaired fasting glucose. The presence of three of these features is considered sufficient to diagnose the syndrome [17].

Inflammation has also been identified as one relevant feature of the metabolic abnormalities found among individuals with MetS [18], which have an increased burden of CVD [19]. Besides the effect on CV morbidity and mortality, the components of MetS have been associated with diabetes. In fact, meta-analyses have clearly shown that MetS increases relative risk of CVD outcomes by about 1.5–2.0 times and of type 2 diabetes by three to five times [20, 21].

Regardless of the fact that the diagnosis of MetS is useful to alert physicians and patients about the risk associated with a sedentary lifestyle and wrong nutritional habits that cause abdominal obesity and its related constellation of metabolic abnormalities, its presence cannot appropriately predict absolute CVD risk [22]. Thus, the risk related to the contribution of MetS to global CVD risk was incorporated in the algorithms through the concept of cardiometabolic risk [22]. In a simple way, the cardiometabolic risk can be defined as the absolute CVD risk determined by traditional risk factors to which we add the additional risk associated with the features of the MetS, thus linking inflammation, obesity (excess visceral/ectopic fat), and insulin resistance to CVD (Fig. 1.1) [18].

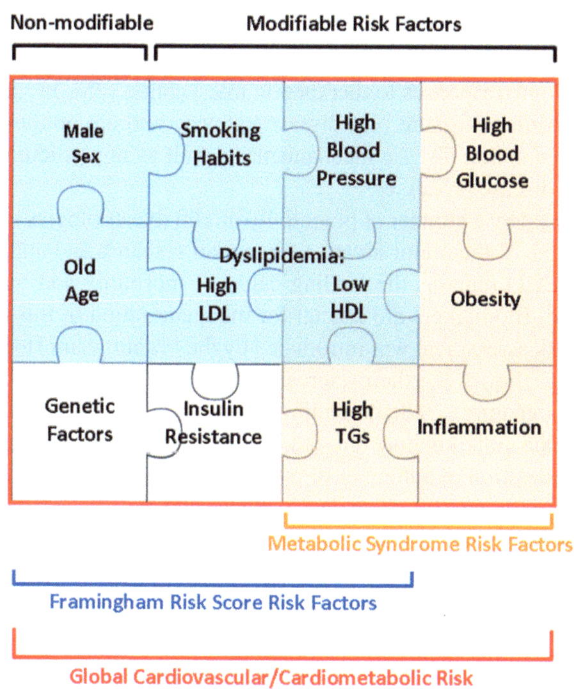

Fig. 1.1 Global cardiovascular/cardiometabolic risk factors (RFs), including the established Framingham Risk Score RFs and the emergent metabolic syndrome RFs related with obesity and inflammation

Established vs. Emergent Biomarkers: Experimental and Clinical Data

Biomarkers and/or risk factors can be either biochemical, physiological, anatomical, or physical, and they can be classified into three broad categories, genetic (including tissue or cellular) biomarkers, imaging biomarkers, and circulating biomarkers, and further into traditional and nontraditional (novel or emergent) risk factors or biomarkers.

The distinction between risk factors and biomarkers for a disease is subtle. The traditional view considers inflammatory biomarkers as risk markers rather than risk factors. A risk factor has a biological role in disease, while a biomarker that is also a risk factor is able to measure a step in pathological processes. A risk marker is statistically associated with the disease, but causality is not an obligatory characteristic of the marker: it is an indirect measure of disease processes and may be a response to other risk factors indeed involved in the pathogenesis, as was previously revised [23, 24].

During the last decades, advances in biomarker research and discovery have allowed remarkable progress in diagnosis and management of several diseases. The US Food and Drug Administration (FDA) defined biomarker as a substance that can be objectively measured as an indicator of normal biologic or pathogenic processes or of pharmacologic responses to therapeutic intervention [25]. In fact, biomarkers provide a more direct measure of a disease pathway and are ubiquitous tools that can aid in understanding disease mechanisms as well as in predicting, diagnosing, and monitoring disease processes.

CVD are caused by a number of potentially modifiable etiologies and risk factors and have been one of the major areas of biomarker research and application, especially because CHD remains the leading cause of morbidity and mortality in the developed world. Biomarkers are crucial for the quantitation of this risk. The concept of global risk assessment was introduced by the Framingham Heart Study more than 50 years ago; however, atherosclerosis is now clearly recognized as having an inflammatory signature, recommending upgrade of risk prediction tools. Understanding the inflammatory cascade in the development of atherosclerosis allows the consideration of a number of inflammatory markers as potentially useful predictors of CVD. Although there is no debate that the inflammatory process is essential to the atherosclerotic lesion, the question raised is whether the inflammatory response characterized by elevated circulating levels of biomarkers is an epiphenomenon or has a causal role. In other words, independently of cholesterol and regulators of blood pressure, could inflammatory biomarkers further report on different aspects of the pathogenic mechanisms underlying the disease?

As stated by Rao et al. [26], for the routine clinical use of a biomarker, several requirements must be accomplished: "1) the ability to control the standardization of the assay and variability of the measurement, 2) consistency in epidemiologic findings from prospective studies with clearly defined endpoints, 3) evidence that the marker adds to risk prediction over and above that already achievable through the use of established risk factors, 4) availability of population norms to guide interpretation of results, 5) generalizability to various population groups, 6) cost-effectiveness—the incremental cost of the test should be justified by a reduction in other costs and the indirect costs of a positive test should not be limiting" [7].

The list of putative biomarkers of inflammation has considerably grown during the last years, accompanying the extensive research on this area of knowledge. In 2003, a Centers for Disease Control and Prevention (CDC)/American Heart Association (AHA) scientific statement on markers of inflammation and CVD considered several inflammatory markers as potentially useful predictors of CVD (adhesion molecules; cytokines; acute-phase reactants, including C-reactive protein [CRP], serum amyloid A protein [SAA], and fibrinogen; white blood cell [WBC] count; and erythrocyte sedimentation rate [ESR]). However, the list of putative biomarkers of inflammation under evaluation during the last years is larger (Table 1.1).

Several other molecules have been associated with inflammation and CVD, but their primary nature is not inflammatory, including oxidative and carbonyl stress compounds; advanced lipoxidation end products (namely, malondialdehyde);

Table 1.1 List of putative biomarkers of inflammation associated with cardiovascular disease

Acute-phase reactants
High-sensitivity C-reactive protein (hsCRP)
Fibrinogen
Serum amyloid A (SAA)
Pro-inflammatory cytokines
Interleukin-1 (IL-1), IL-6, IL-18
Tumor necrosis factor alpha (TNF-α)
Interferon gamma (IFN-γ)
CD40/CD40 ligand
Anti-inflammatory cytokines
Interleukin (IL)-4, IL-10
Transforming growth factor (TGF-β)
Adiponectin
Other adipocytokines (leptin, resistin, visfatin)
Cell adhesion molecules
E-selectin, P-selectin
Intercellular cell adhesion molecule-1 (ICAM-1)
Vascular cell adhesion molecule-1 (VCAM-1)
Platelet endothelial cell adhesion molecule-1 (PECAM-1)
Chemokines
Interleukin-8 (IL-8)
Migration inhibitory factor (MIF)
Monocyte chemoattractant-1 (MCP-1)
Other molecules/mediators of inflammation
Matrix metalloproteinases (MMPs)
Myeloperoxidase (MPO)
Myeloid-related protein (MRP) 8/14
White blood cell (WBC) count
Erythrocyte sedimentation rate (ESR)

advanced glycosylation end products (AGEs), such as plasma F2α-isoprostanes, advanced oxidation protein products, pentosidine, and carboxymethyl lysine; hemostatic and endothelial injury/dysfunction factors, including plasminogen activator inhibitor type 1, von Willebrand factor, and asymmetric dimethylarginine; homocysteine; lipid-associated markers, i.e., oxidized LDL and antibody to oxidized LDL, small dense LDL particles, lipoprotein (a), lipoprotein-associated phospholipase A2 (Lp-PLA2); heat shock protein (HSPs); and RANTES (regulated on activation, normal T cell expressed and secreted), among others.

Regarding clinical utility of putative inflammatory biomarkers of CV risk, it is important to consider some questions: does the biomarker add any information to that available from existing and well-established risk factors? Is it a suitable analyte? Is it stable in terms of diet influences and variations intra- and inter-day? Preferably, the biomarker should provide additional and independent information on cardiovascular risk; it should be easy to measure using standardized commercial assays with low variability and reasonably priced and not requiring specialized plasma collection or assay techniques. CRP has emerged as a robust, yet controversial clinical marker, since some of the previous requirements are accomplished.

This chapter starts exploring the most relevant data available and controversies and doubts concerning the putative use of CRP as a clinical biomarker of CV risk. Other molecule candidates to act as inflammatory biomarkers will be also debated.

High-Sensitivity C-Reactive Protein

High-sensitivity C-reactive protein (hsCRP) was first discovered in 1930, but its link to CHD was reported more than 60 years later. hsCRP is an acute-phase reactant mainly produced in hepatocytes in response to several cytokines, including IL-6 released from activated leukocytes in response to infection or trauma and from vascular SMCs during atherosclerosis lesion evolution. The role of CRP in atherosclerotic plaque formation is complex, acting in many cells involved in the process (Fig. 1.2) [27]. Although previous reports suggested a role of CRP as a surrogate of the underlying inflammatory process of atherothrombosis, accumulating evidence from in vitro and in vivo studies in clinical and experimental models robustly indicate a role of CRP as a proatherogenic factor [27–30].

In brief, CRP induces endothelial cell activation and dysfunction by several distinct activities, including directly binding with highly atherogenic oxidized LDL-C (oxLDL); increasing adhesion molecules (VCAM-1, ICAM-1, E-selectin, MCP-1); decreasing eNOS, prostacyclin, and tPA; impairing endothelial progenitor cell (EPC) number and function; and increasing pro-inflammatory cytokines and other important mediators of endothelial lesion (such as PAI-1, IL-8, CD40/CD40L, MMP-1, and ET-1) underlying atherosclerosis; in addition, it facilitates monocyte adhesion and transmigration into the vessel wall, a critical early step in the atherosclerotic process, and promotes other important modifications on monocytes (increasing tissue factor, superoxide, and myeloperoxidase contents, decreasing

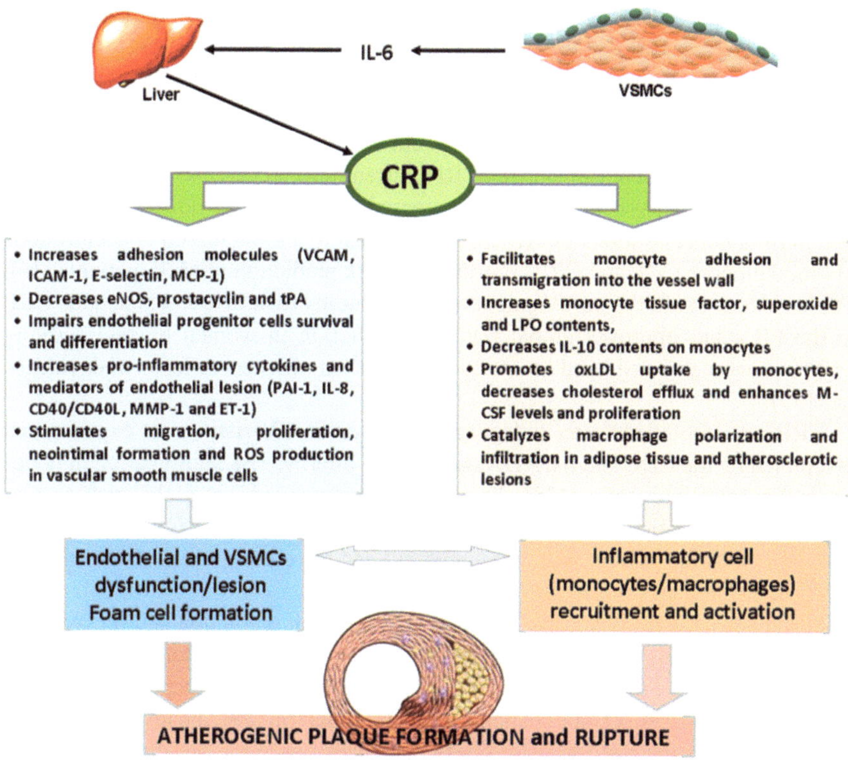

Fig. 1.2 Potential mechanisms of C-reactive protein (CRP) involvement in the pathogenesis of atherosclerotic plaque formation and rupture. While it remains uncertain whether CRP is directly involved in the pathogenesis of atherosclerosis or it is just a surrogate marker (an epiphenomenon) of other processes, several lines of evidence have been suggesting that CRP is localized within atherosclerotic lesions and exerts pro-inflammatory and proatherogenic effects

IL-10 amounts, promoting oxLDL uptake, decreasing cholesterol efflux, and enhancing macrophage colony-stimulating factor [M-CSF] levels and proliferation); CRP also catalyzes macrophage polarization, which is a pro-inflammatory trigger in plaque deposition, leading to macrophage infiltration of both adipose tissue and atherosclerotic lesions [27–30].

Several lines of evidence have indicated that inflammation plays a central role in all stages of the atherothrombotic process. In clinical terms, translation of the atherosclerosis inflammatory hypothesis to practice has been based on observational evidence linking inflammatory biomarkers to the risk of future vascular events, namely, using hsCRP [31–33]. In fact, large-scale prospective studies demonstrate that CRP strongly and independently predicts adverse CV events, including MI, ischemic stroke, and sudden cardiac death [14, 33, 34]. The inclusion of CRP to classical cholesterol screening improves CV risk prediction independently of LDL-C, suggesting that increased CRP may identify asymptomatic individuals at high risk for future events, despite average cholesterol concentrations [33]. Furthermore,

CRP concentration monitoring adds relevant prognostic information on CV risk at all LDL-C concentrations, but also at all levels of the FRS [33, 34]. As shown in the meta-analysis of Kaptoge et al., the magnitude of CV risk associated with a one-standard-deviation increase in hsCRP levels is at least as large as that associated with a one-standard-deviation increase in either total cholesterol or blood pressure [35]. Additionally, increased plasma CRP concentrations correlate with the components of MetS, such as central obesity, increased plasma triglyceride concentrations, low plasma concentrations of HDL-C, hypertension, and increased concentrations of blood glucose [33], and CRP contributes to risk prediction of MetS patients [36]. This evidence led to the development of the Reynolds Risk Score, which adds CRP to the FRS and improves global CV risk prediction in women by reclassifying >50 % of women considered at intermediate risk into higher- or lower-risk categories [37].

CRP was classified as an independent marker of CV risk by an expert panel assembled by the CDC and the AHA, as a way to improve risk stratification in populations' primary prevention [38]. The panel recommended that global risk prediction in asymptomatic individuals deemed at intermediate risk for CVD by classical risk factors should include CRP measurement and the cutoff points of <1 mg/L for low-risk and >3 mg/L for high-risk individuals.

Further than being used as an adjunctive tool in risk prediction and reclassification, there is interest in using hsCRP levels to select patients for statin initiation and to tailor intensity of therapy. Statins reduce hsCRP in an LDL-independent manner, and the benefits are superior in patients with inflammation [39]; the lower the hsCRP levels, the lower the risk [40, 41]. These evidences raised the question of whether patients that do not meet criteria for statin prescription (given the low/average LDL-C concentrations) would benefit from that medication if they had hsCRP > 2 mg/L, indicative of an enhanced inflammatory response, thus suggesting that statins could have a dual influence: reduction of LDL-C levels and direct anti-inflammatory effects. These questions/hypotheses were the basis for the JUPITER trial (Justification for the Use of Statins in Prevention: an Intervention Trial Evaluating Rosuvastatin) [42], which enrolled 17,802 men and women with no evidence of CV disease and average or low LDL-C contents, for testing the putative benefit of rosuvastatin (20 mg po daily) treatment. JUPITER trial showed a major reduction in CV events (54 % in MI and 51 % in ischemic stroke) and in all-cause mortality (20 %), as well as in need for bypass surgery or angioplasty (46 %), with an overall 44 % relative risk reduction for the primary endpoint of major arterial vascular events. Results were identical between several subpopulations in all ethnic groups, including women vs. men, elderly, as well as with and without arterial hypertension, obesity, or MetS [42–44]. As recently commended [45], JUPITER trial also showed that there was a significant reduction in venous thromboembolism (43 %), and the maximum levels of risk reduction were found in those who achieved low hsCRP levels. Magnitude of hsCRP reduction could not be predicted on the basis of the magnitude of LDL-C reduction, and the reduction of absolute risk of events for both the rosuvastatin-treated and placebo-treated (control) groups was greater among those with higher levels of CRP at study entry, an effect not observed for LDL-C. Genetic determinants of rosuvastatin-induced LDL-C reduction were found to differ from the genetic determinants of rosuvastatin-induced CRP reduction, altogether suggesting that at least part of the benefits of statin therapy were due to anti-inflammatory effects independent of LDL-C reduction. All those strong evidences coming from JUPITER trial, including the smaller number needed to treat (NNT) found for subjects with low LDL-C levels and elevated hsCRP concentrations (when compared with primary prevention patients under treatment of dyslipidemia or arterial hypertension) [46], had impacted the spectrum of patients candidate for statin therapy according to the FDA, as well as to other several national authorities, now including patients with elevated hsCRP levels and at least one additional risk factor, independently of high or average LDL-C levels.

Despite several strong indications coming from that trial, highlighting a statin benefit that goes beyond the effect on LDL-C reduction, additional studies were recommended to clearly test the hypothesis that directly targeting inflammation will improve vascular outcomes. The Canakinumab Anti-inflammatory Thrombosis Outcomes Study (CANTOS) and the Cardiovascular Inflammation Reduction Trial (CIRT) have recently started and will evaluate, respectively, a human monoclonal antibody that targets human interleukin-1β (IL-1β) and low-dose methotrexate, in order to reduce cardiovascular event rates, due to direct anti-inflammatory effects [47, 48]. The results of these trials are expected with great curiosity, as they could be essential to define new algorithms to improve CV risk prediction and to gather information that could serve as basis to define new drugs targeting the machinery of inflammation.

Emergent Biomarkers

Other Acute-Phase Reactants

Serum amyloid A (SAA) protein and fibrinogen, like CRP, are acute-phase reactants generated downstream of IL-6 in the liver, as part of the acute-phase response, reflecting the intensity of cytokine activation.

Fibrinogen

Fibrinogen influences endothelial function, thrombosis, and inflammation and has been indicated as an independent variable contributing to CV risk. In brief, fibrinogen forms the substrate for thrombin (leading to platelet aggregation), modulates endothelial function, and promotes SMC proliferation and migration [49]. Several epidemiologic studies demonstrate that fibrinogen concentrations predict future risk of MI and stroke. However, it seems to be a less potent predictor of CV events than CRP [50]. Whether or not fibrinogen is causally involved in atherothrombogenesis remains to be elucidated.

Serum Amyloid A (SAA)

SAA protein, like CRP, is an acute-phase protein synthesized in the liver in response to infection, inflammation, injury, or stress. It has been linked to atherosclerosis, namely, because it is secreted as the predominant apolipoprotein on plasma HDL cholesterol particles, where it seems to replace apolipoprotein A-I, thus changing HDL-mediated cholesterol delivery to cells [51].

The more rapid response of SAA than other nonspecific inflammatory markers, such as CRP, has suggested that it could be a better marker of disease. SAA has also been shown to be a predictor of CV events [52]. However, some studies suggest that this relationship may be dependent on other risk factors [32], indicating that the independent predictive value of SAA for CAD and CV events remains unclear, deserving further studies.

Cytokines

Cytokines are key in regulating inflammatory and immune responses and have a pivotal role in controlling the innate and the adaptive immunity. Pathogenesis of atherosclerosis involves a complex interplay between cytokines, chemokines, and adhesion molecules, leading to monocyte infiltration and multiple other leukocyte responses within the arterial wall. A variety of plasma inflammatory markers have been shown to predict future CV risk. In addition, they may be useful for risk stratification and also to identify patients who might benefit from targeted therapy. Cytokines are classified according to their pro- or anti-inflammatory activities. The balance between pro- and anti-inflammatory cytokines has emerged as a major determinant of plaque stability [53].

Pro-inflammatory Cytokines

Several inflammatory cytokines have also been investigated as markers of CV risk, including TNF-α, IL-6, and CD40/CD40 ligand.

Tumor Necrosis Factor Alpha (TNF-α)

TNF-α is a cytokine primarily produced by macrophages, endothelial cells, and SMCs of atherosclerotic arteries and has been shown to have several pro-inflammatory properties, including induction of expression of cellular adhesion molecules, surface leukocyte adhesion molecules, chemokines, other cytokines, and growth factors, as well as proangiogenic activity [54]. TNF-α activities affect atherosclerotic process and have been implicated in metabolic disorders, such as obesity and insulin resistance [54, 55]. Increased plasma concentrations of TNF-α have been associated with increased risk of CV events, namely, in stable patients after MI, as it was demonstrated in the Cholesterol and Recurrent Events (CARE) trial [56].

Interleukin-6 (IL-6)

IL-6 is produced by hepatocytes, endothelial cells, fibroblasts, phagocytes, neutrophils, and lymphocytes, among other cell types. This pleiotropic cytokine has a broad range of functions and regulates several cellular processes, including growth, differentiation, angiogenesis, and healing. The precise role of IL-6 in the evolution of atherosclerosis lesions remains uncertain, but several important activities/effects of IL-6 have been described, namely, in ApoE knockout mice, including stimulation of synthesis and secretion of CRP and enhancement of fatty lesion development [57]. Increased levels of IL-6 seem to be predictive of future CV events, as suggested in the Physicians' Health Study (PHS) [58].

CD40/CD40 Ligand

CD40 ligand (CD40L) is a transmembrane protein of the TNF family that links to its receptor (CD40) and has a role in the inflammatory processes underlying atherosclerosis, plaque destabilization, and thrombosis. In fact, CD40/CD40L, expressed in a variety of immune and vascular cells, regulates platelet-dependent responses that contribute to atherothrombosis, activate endothelial cells, and in vitro promote expression of adhesion molecules, pro-inflammatory cytokines, and chemokines [59]. Soluble CD40L levels have been indicated as predictive of CV events (MI and stroke) and death in some populations [60].

Anti-inflammatory Cytokines

Interleukin-4 (IL-4) and IL-10

IL-4 and IL-10 are pleiotropic cytokines produced by Th2 lymphocytes and by other types of immune cells that have been associated with anti-inflammatory activities, mostly in mouse models of atherosclerosis. While decreased IL-10 levels have been reported in patients with acute CV events [61], the association of IL-4 levels with CVD is debatable as IL-4 may also play a role in atherosclerosis through induction of inflammatory responses (it is worth to say that increased IL-4 levels were found in patients with CAD) [62].

Transforming Growth Factor Beta (TGF-β)

TGF-β is a potent anti-inflammatory cytokine that plays a pivotal role in the maintenance of normal blood vessel wall architecture and protects against vulnerability to atherosclerosis. TGF-β isoforms 1, 2, and 3 are mainly expressed by SMCs and modulate vascular development and remodeling and determine the extent to which developing atherosclerotic lesions are stabilized [63]. Decreased levels of TGF-β1, as well as genetic polymorphisms and defective TGF-β signaling, have been reported in patients with CVD [64, 65].

Adiponectin

Adiponectin is an adipocytokine produced by adipocytes that exerts anti-inflammatory and antiatherogenic effects, having a protective role in CV terms [66]. It reduces TNF-α-stimulated expression of E-selectin, NF-κB, VCAM-1, and IL-8 and regulates monocyte adhesion to endothelium and endothelial nitric oxide synthase (eNOS) activity. Adiponectin also has insulin-sensitizing effects, and its secretion diminishes as adipose tissue mass increases. It is suggested that adiponectin contributes to the relationship between obesity, insulin resistance, and CV disease. Its concentrations are inversely associated with CVD incidence in most of the studies. In the PHS, there was a robust inverse relationship between total adiponectin and incident CHD, even after adjustment for traditional risk factors, while high levels of adiponectin have been associated with lower risk for CV events [67, 68].

These observations suggest that there is promise for the application of adiponectin and other cytokines as predictors of CVD risk. However, since the associations are complex, a more complete understanding of the exact role played by these emergent biomarkers in disease's pathophysiology is required, as well as stronger evidences from larger clinical studies without confounding factors and after proper adjustment for traditional risk factors.

Cell Adhesion Molecules

Due to their central role in the recruitment of inflammatory cells to the site of atheroma development, the cell adhesion molecules (CAMs) are promising candidates to reflect underlying vascular inflammation. E-selectin, vascular cell adhesion molecule-1 (VCAM-1), and intercellular cell adhesion molecule-1 (ICAM-1) are all members of the cellular adhesion molecule family, each having a plasma-soluble form, which can serve as a surrogate marker for increased expression of CAMs on vascular endothelial cells, reflecting inflammation and activation of endothelial cells [69].

E-Selectin

E-selectin is the most interesting form of the selectin family, which also includes L and P selectins. E-selectin promotes the interaction between endothelial cells, where it is expressed, to leukocytes. While increased E-selectin levels have been observed in some studies with CVD populations, other reports showed divergent results; at the moment, the prognostic value of E-selectin remains to be clearly defined [69, 70].

Intercellular Cell Adhesion Molecule-1 (ICAM-1)

ICAM-1 mediates attachment of circulating leukocytes to the endothelium and their subsequent transmigration and accumulation in the arterial intima, thus promoting progression of atherosclerosis. The circulating soluble form of ICAM-1, which is expressed on the surface of endothelial cells, leukocytes, and SMCs in response to a variety of stimuli (such as shear stress and pro-inflammatory cytokines), is released from endothelial cell membranes and may be viewed as a marker of atherosclerosis. Increased levels of ICAM-1 have been shown to predict future CV events and are associated with death due to CV events in distinct populations [71, 72].

Vascular Cell Adhesion Molecule-1 (VCAM-1)

VCAM-1 expression in vessels is increased when endothelial cells are stimulated by cytokines (namely, TNF-α and IL-1), facilitating adhesion and migration of leukocytes across the endothelial barrier. sICAM-l is viewed as a general marker of a pro-inflammatory status and correlates with CRP in primary prevention studies. While ICAM-1 predicts symptomatic disease in healthy individuals, VCAM-1 seems to be a better marker of the extent and severity of atherosclerosis in patients with established disease. VCAM-1 has been reported to predict future cardiovascular events in patients with CAD and CHD [71, 73] and proved to be a better predictor than ICAM and E-selectin in a study that evaluated these three cell adhesion molecules [73].

E-selectin, VCAM-1, and ICAM-1 could be viewed as markers of inflammation and activation of endothelial cells, but their prognostic value remains unclear, deserving further elucidation.

Chemokines

Chemokines are pro-inflammatory chemotactic cytokines present in circulation and in atherosclerotic lesions and cause leukocyte migration into vascular-inflamed tissue, being also involved in SMC migration and growth and platelet activation [74].

Interleukin-8 (IL-8)

IL-8 is mainly produced by monocytes and macrophages and acts as a chemoattractant for neutrophils and T lymphocytes. While most of the current knowledge was obtained from experimental animal studies, clinical data showed that IL-8 might have a predictive value for CV events, namely, in patients presenting with acute MI [75].

Migration Inhibitory Factor (MIF)

MIF is expressed in a wide variety of tissues, where it is able to promote the synthesis of other pro-inflammatory mediators. During the progression of atherosclerosis, MIF is overexpressed in endothelial cells, SMCs, and macrophages [76]. Preclinical and clinical data have been showing divergent data, but increased circulating levels of MIF were associated to future CV events in patients with stable CAD and type 2 diabetes mellitus, even after adjusting for the traditional risk factors [77].

Monocyte Chemoattractant-1 (MCP-1)

MCP-1 is one of the key chemokines that regulate migration and infiltration of monocytes and macrophages and appears to play a relevant role in atherosclerotic lesions. Elevated levels of MCP-1 have been suggested as direct markers of inflammation for populations of CVD risk [78].

Other Molecules

Matrix Metalloproteinases (MMPs)

MMPs are a family of endopeptidases predominantly expressed in macrophages but also in vascular SMCs, lymphocytes, and endothelial cells, playing a role in vascular remodeling, progression of atherosclerosis, and plaque destabilization [79]. By degrading the extracellular matrix, MPPs promote increment of plaque vulnerability when submitted to mechanical stresses, thus increasing risk of acute CV events. In fact, increased levels of MMPs were found in distinct risk populations, namely, in those with acute coronary syndromes [80].

Myeloperoxidase (MPO)

MPO is a heme protein mainly secreted by activated neutrophils and monocytes, which has also been found in human plaques and exerts proatherogenic effects, including oxidation of LDL and reduction of NO bioavailability [81]. Elevated levels of MPO have been indicated as an independent predictor of mortality in acute MI patients and of future CV events, even after correction for traditional risk factors and CRP; however, it seems to be a weaker predictor than these established CV risk factors and CRP [82, 83].

Unanswered Questions and Challenges

The revolution in the understanding of the pathophysiology of atherosclerosis has focused interest on inflammation and provided new insight into mechanisms of disease. Several lines of evidence illustrate the remarkable data that associate inflammation with risk of future CV events and emphasize the pivotal relevance of inflammatory mechanisms in determining plaque vulnerability. Clinical application of the concept that inflammation is crucial in the initiation and progression of atherosclerosis illustrates the translation of basic science understanding to clinical practice.

During the last years, several putative biomarkers of inflammation have been tentatively adopted to improve diagnostic capacity, to monitor disease activity and efficacy of therapy, as well as to improve prognosis. However, evaluation of clinical use of biomarkers in the context of atherosclerotic CV disease requires considerable attention, starting from proper distinction between risk factor and risk marker, which depends whether (risk factor) or not (biomarker) it has a causal role in the pathology. Additionally, the putative utility of the biomarker should be clearly established, defining if it will be useful for risk stratification of healthy individuals or diseased populations, if it could be used per se or in addition to traditional accepted risk factors, or if it could be used to monitor efficacy of therapy. These questions will determine the type of validation needed. Before a novel marker reaches clinical application, important conditions must be met: there should be robust data coming from several large-scale prospective studies; the marker must improve knowledge upon traditional risk evaluation; there should be a standardized assay to its feasible quantification, and it should potentially assist in therapeutic interventions.

Although the circulating concentrations of several inflammatory mediators correlate with increased CV risk or were able to predict future events, few have been able to be considered as really candidates for clinical use. Despite the controversies, hsCRP has been viewed as the strongest candidate to clinically act as a biomarker. hsCRP has proved to be robust because it is a stable protein (analyte), with a standardized and high-sensitivity assay, it has minor diurnal variations and a long plasma half-life, and it is independent of food intake. One of the major problems is that elevated levels of hsCRP, despite strongly associated with risk, do not allow to infer directly the presence of a disease, but of an inflammatory state, acting as a biomarker rather than a risk factor. The causality can only be considered after properly excluding the contribution of confounders. A wide collection of studies shows that epidemiologic associations between hsCRP and CVD outcomes are independent of other risk factors. However, several of them have not properly adjusted all the modifiable (obesity, insulin resistance, or physical inactivity) and non-modifiable (genetic or ethnic characteristics) risk factors, which is obviously relevant, because several risk factors for atherosclerosis, such as smoking habits, obesity, insulin resistance, diabetes, or dyslipidemia, are themselves associated with increased inflammation.

Emerging evidence has shown a strong relationship between hsCRP and various characteristics of MetS. The addition of hsCRP measurement to the actual definition of MetS may help in identifying patients at high risk for future diabetes and CVD. Further research is required to clarify the precise role of hsCRP in MetS pathogenesis and whether it is able to improve prediction of CV events in patients with elevated hsCRP concentrations.

Accumulated evidence of improved CV risk prediction using hsCRP levels independently of LDL-C led to the development of the Reynolds Risk Score, which adds hsCRP to the FRS and improves global CV risk prediction in women by reclassifying up to 50 % of subjects considered at intermediate risk into higher- or lower-risk categories. An expert panel assembled by CDC and AHA has recommended that global risk prediction in asymptomatic individuals deemed at intermediate risk for

CVD by classical risk factors should include hsCRP measurement using the cutoff points of <1 mg/L for low-risk and >3 mg/L for high-risk individuals.

If hsCRP is a risk factor with a causal role, interventions targeted towards lowering its levels should improve outcomes. JUPITER study showed a clear benefit of aggressive statin (rosuvastatin) therapy in patients with hsCRP greater than 2 mg/L that do not meet formal criteria for statin prescription (given the low/average LDL-C concentrations). The remarkable reduction in CV events and in all-cause mortality, among several other positive indications, in the JUPITER trial, suggested that at least part of the benefits of statin therapy were due to anti-inflammatory effects independent of LDL-C reduction. That strong evidence coming from the trial had impacted on the spectrum of statin clinical usage according to the FDA, as well as several national authorities, now considering for treating patients with elevated hsCRP levels and at least one additional risk factor, independently of high or average LDL-C levels. Two clinical trials (CANTOS and CIRT) are ongoing, aiming to test the hypothesis that directly targeting inflammation will improve vascular outcomes and the results might bring new light on the issue.

With the exception of hsCRP, until now, none of the emerging/novel inflammation biomarkers for CV risk has demonstrated additive value to the FRS, and few have available commercial assays that achieve adequate levels of standardization and accuracy for clinical use. Like CRP, SAA and fibrinogen are acute-phase reactants that seem to be involved in several steps of atherosclerosis mechanisms, despite that an undoubtedly causal role in atherothrombogenesis remains to be elucidated. In addition, fibrinogen seems to be a less potent predictor of CV events than hsCRP, and the predictive value of SAA for CAD and CV events seems to be dependent on other risk factors, deserving further research.

The balance between pro- and anti-inflammatory cytokines may be important for risk stratification and also to identify patients who might benefit from targeted therapy. Measurement of pro-inflammatory (namely, IL-6, IL-1, TNF-α, and INF-γ) and anti-inflammatory cytokines (namely, IL-4, IL-10, TGF-β, and adiponectin) may be useful for indicating the complex interplay between inflammatory and anti-inflammatory processes. Despite preclinical and clinical evidences suggesting that pro-inflammatory cytokines (namely, TNF-α, IL-6, and sCD40L), but also INF-γ and IL-1, have a role in atherosclerosis development and that their levels could be predictive of future CVD events and CV deaths, more data are needed, in order to validate these molecules as biomarkers of CVD. The clinical utility of adiponectin is based on its strong epidemiologic relationships with obesity, inflammation, and diabetes, strengthened by its established biological actions in blood vessels and immune cells. Adiponectin levels have been widely evaluated as epidemiologic markers of diabetes and CVD risk, and increased concentrations of adiponectin are being studied as indicators of treatment need, as predictors of response to therapy, and as markers of therapeutic effectiveness, in order to feasibly translate adiponectin measurements into clinical practice.

E-selectin, VCAM-1, and ICAM-1, all belonging to the cellular adhesion molecule family, have been tested as markers of early onset of inflammation, but their prognostic value remains uncertain. VCAM-1 seems to be unable to act as risk factor in healthy individuals but as strong predictor of risk in patients.

The role of chemokines (including IL-8, MCP-1, and MIF) as biomarkers remains also unclear. While IL-8 and MCP-1 have shown ability to act as markers of inflammation in subpopulations of CVD-diagnosed patients, MIF seems to show ability to predict future CV events in patients with stable CAD or type 2 diabetes. MMPs may be useful for prognosis in patients with ACS, while elevated MPO levels have been suggested to predict future risk of CAD in healthy subjects, but for both of them, available data are insufficient to dispose of a direct clinical application.

Studies including a larger number of patients are needed to confirm some data already available. However, some strategies must be previously considered to be successful, such as include serial determinations in protocols (and not only baseline measurements) and recruit preferably patients with preexisting CAD or ACS, instead of healthy populations. In addition, the quality of the trials and the power of the evidence will depend on the evaluation of the relationship between the concentrations of these molecules and the degree of atherosclerosis and plaque instability, which is better estimated using new technical approaches, namely, molecular imaging.

Due to the complexities of CVD pathogenesis, a single biomarker cannot be used to estimate absolute risk of future CV events. Furthermore, particular biomarkers are more suited for prognosis of particular events and for a given stage of a given CVD. It should also be recognized that the biological functions of many biomarkers may overlap. Therefore, they should be selected for a specific stage of a given disease, and a particular biomarker should not be considered in isolation. Simultaneous measurements of disease appropriate biomarkers over time can provide a more detailed picture of the specific nature of the CV event.

It is also important to underscore that the lack of value as a biomarker does not exclude an important pathogenic role of these molecules in atherogenesis and plaque destabilization and, accordingly, does not negate the potential value as novel targets for therapy in atherosclerotic disorders.

Further studies, both in progress and on the horizon, will help to evaluate the role of novel and emerging biomarkers in the clinical management of atherosclerosis and targeting of therapies. Until then, while measurement of inflammatory biomarkers is a valuable adjunct to CVD risk assessment, the emphasis should not digress from lowering the burden of conventional modifiable risk factors.

Take-Home Messages

- Even though conventional risk factors in the FRS account for most of the risk of CV events, a substantial percentage of subjects die from CHD. In addition, many of those events occur in patients treated with statins and presenting with cholesterol levels below population average. Thus, an improved ability to predict CV risk and decrease the high level of residual risk of further CV events is mandatory.
- A major shift in the paradigm of our understanding of atherosclerosis pathogenesis has been seen in the last decade, which is now recognized as having a clear inflammatory signature, since inflammatory mechanisms play a crucial role in all

phases of the disease, from initial recruitment of circulating leucocytes to the arterial wall to eventual rupture of the unstable plaque.
- The ominous presence of inflammation in atherosclerosis allows the consideration of a number of emergent biomarkers as potentially useful tools to help in identifying patients at high risk for future CV events, including acute-phase reactants, pro- and anti-inflammatory cytokines, cell adhesion molecules, chemokines, as well as other mediators involved in the pathogenesis of atherosclerosis.
- While experimental and/or clinical data have been shown the possibility of several emergent biomarkers to have predictive value in determining future CV events and/or death, until now only hsCRP has demonstrated additive value to the FRS. Therefore, an expert panel assembled by the CDC and the AHA recommended that global risk prediction in asymptomatic individuals deemed at intermediate risk for CVD by classical risk factors should include hsCRP measurement and the cutoff points of <1 mg/L for low-risk and >3 mg/L for high-risk individuals.
- Further studies, some of them already ongoing and others on the horizon, will define the precise value of all these novel/emerging biomarkers of inflammation in the clinical management of CVD risk prediction and therapy.

Acknowledgments/Support The authors thank Portuguese Foundation for Science and Technology (FCT), COMPETE-FEDER and POPH/FSE, through the following support: PTDC/SAU-TOX/114253/2009, UID/NEU/04539/2013 (CNC.IBILI).

References

1. Stavitsky AB. The innate immune response to infection, toxins and trauma evolved into networks of interactive, defensive, reparative, regulatory, injurious and pathogenic pathways. Mol Immunol. 2007;44(11):2787–99.
2. Roda JM, Eubank TD. Chapter 2: The cellular component of chronic inflammation. In: Roy S, Bagchi D, Raychaudhuri SP, editors. Chronic inflammation: molecular pathophysiology, nutritional and therapeutic interventions. Boca Raton: CRC Press, Taylor & Francis Group; 2013. p. 21–33.
3. World Health Organization. Global status report on non-communicable diseases 2010. Geneva: World Health Organization; 2011.
4. Ghazalpour A, Doss S, Yang X, Aten J, Toomey EM, Van Nas A, et al. Thematic review series: the pathogenesis of atherosclerosis. Toward a biological network for atherosclerosis. J Lipid Res. 2004;45(10):1793–805.
5. Khot UN, Khot MB, Bajzer CT, Sapp SK, Ohman EM, Brener SJ, et al. Prevalence of conventional risk factors in patients with coronary heart disease. JAMA. 2003;290(7):898–904.
6. Smith Jr SC. Current and future directions of cardiovascular risk prediction. Am J Cardiol. 2006;97(2A):28A–32.
7. Baigent C, Keech A, Kearney PM, Blackwell L, Buck G, Pollicino C, et al. Efficacy and safety of cholesterol lowering treatment: prospective meta-analysis of data from 90,056 participants in 14 randomised trials of statins. Lancet. 2005;366(9493):1267–78.
8. Cannon CP, Braunwald E, McCabe CH, Rader DJ, Rouleau JL, Belder R, et al. Intensive versus moderate lipid lowering with statins after acute coronary syndromes. N Engl J Med. 2004;350(15):1495–504.

9. Ross R. Atherosclerosis — an inflammatory disease. N Engl J Med. 1999;340(2):115–26.
10. Shah PK. Mechanisms of plaque vulnerability and rupture. J Am Coll Cardiol. 2003;41(4 Suppl 1):S15–22.
11. Nissen SE, Yock P. Intravascular ultrasound: novel pathophysiological insights and current clinical applications. Circulation. 2001;103(4):604–16.
12. Libby P, Ridker PM, Hansson GK. Progress and challenges in translating the biology of atherosclerosis. Nature. 2011;473(7347):317–25.
13. Galkina E, Ley K. Immune and inflammatory mechanisms of atherosclerosis. Annu Rev Immunol. 2009;27:165–97.
14. Pai JK, Pischon T, Ma J, Manson JE, Hankinson SE, Joshipura K, et al. Inflammatory markers and the risk of coronary heart disease in men and women. N Engl J Med. 2004;351(25):2599–610.
15. Libby P, Aikawa M. Stabilization of atherosclerotic plaques: new mechanisms and clinical targets. Nat Med. 2002;8(11):1257–62.
16. Alberti KG, Zimmet P, Shaw J. The metabolic syndrome – a new worldwide definition. Lancet. 2005;366(9491):1059–62.
17. Expert Panel on Detection, Evaluation, and Treatment of High Blood Cholesterol in Adults: Executive Summary of the Third Report of the National Cholesterol Education Program (NCEP) Expert Panel on Detection, Evaluation, and Treatment of High Blood Cholesterol in Adults (Adult Treatment Panel III.) JAMA. 2001;285(19):2486–97.
18. Després JP. Abdominal obesity and cardiovascular disease: is inflammation the missing link? Can J Cardiol. 2012;28(6):642–52.
19. Haffner S, Cassells HB. Metabolic syndrome – a new risk factor of coronary heart disease? Diabetes Obes Metab. 2003;5(6):359–70.
20. Galassi A, Reynolds K, He J. Metabolic syndrome and risk of cardiovascular disease: a meta-analysis. Am J Med. 2006;119(10):812–9.
21. Gami AS, Witt BJ, Howard DE, Erwin PJ, Gami LA, Somers VK, et al. Metabolic syndrome and risk of incident cardiovascular events and death: a systematic review and meta-analysis of longitudinal studies. J Am Coll Cardiol. 2007;49(4):403–14.
22. Després JP, Lemieux I. Abdominal obesity and metabolic syndrome. Nature. 2006;444(7121):881–7.
23. Vasan RS. Biomarkers of cardiovascular disease: molecular basis and practical considerations. Circulation. 2006;113(19):2335–62.
24. Ge Y, Wang TJ. Circulating, imaging, and genetic biomarkers in cardiovascular risk prediction. Trends Cardiovasc Med. 2011;21(4):105–12.
25. Biomarkers Definitions Working Group. Biomarkers and surrogate endpoints: preferred definitions and conceptual framework. Clin Pharmacol Ther. 2001;69(3):89–95.
26. Rao M, Jaber BL, Balakrishnan VS. Inflammatory biomarkers and cardiovascular risk: association or cause and effect? Semin Dial. 2006;19(2):129–35.
27. Devaraj S, Singh U, Jialal I. The evolving role of C-reactive protein in atherothrombosis. Clin Chem. 2009;55(2):229–38.
28. Verma S, Szmitko PE, Ridker PM. C-reactive protein comes of age. Nat Clin Pract Cardiovasc Med. 2005;2(1):29–36.
29. Verma S, Devaraj S, Jialal I. Is C-reactive protein an innocent bystander or proatherogenic culprit? C-reactive protein promotes atherothrombosis. Circulation. 2006;113(17):2135–50.
30. Devaraj S, Yun JM, Adamson G, Galvez J, Jialal I. C-reactive protein impairs the endothelial glycocalyx resulting in endothelial dysfunction. Cardiovasc Res. 2009;84(3):479–84.
31. Libby P, Ridker PM, Hansson GK. Inflammation in atherosclerosis: from pathophysiology to practice. J Am Coll Cardiol. 2009;54(23):2129–38.
32. Ridker PM, Hennekens CH, Buring JE, Rifai N. C-reactive protein and other markers of inflammation in the prediction of cardiovascular disease in women. N Engl J Med. 2000;342(12):836–43.
33. Ridker PM, Rifai N, Rose L, Buring JE, Cook NR. Comparison of C-reactive protein and low-density lipoprotein cholesterol levels in the prediction of first cardiovascular events. N Engl J Med. 2002;347(20):1557–65.

34. Koenig W, Lowel H, Baumert J, Meisinger C. C-reactive protein modulates risk prediction based on the Framingham Score: implications for future risk assessment: results from a large cohort study in southern Germany. Circulation. 2004;109(11):1349–53.
35. Kaptoge S, Di Angelantonio E, Lowe G, Pepys MB, Thompson SG, Collins R, et al. C-reactive protein concentration and risk of coronary heart disease, stroke, and mortality: an individual participant meta-analysis. Lancet. 2010;375(9709):132–40.
36. Ridker PM, Buring JE, Cook NR, Rifai N. C-reactive protein, the metabolic syndrome, and risk of incident cardiovascular events: an 8-year follow-up of 14 719 initially healthy American women. Circulation. 2003;107(3):391–7.
37. Ridker PM, Buring JE, Rifai N, Cook NR. Development and validation of improved algorithms for the assessment of global cardiovascular risk in women: the Reynolds risk score. JAMA. 2007;297(6):611–9.
38. Pearson TA, Mensah GA, Alexander RW, Anderson JL, Cannon 3rd RO, Criqui M, et al. Markers of inflammation and cardiovascular disease: application to clinical and public health practice: a statement for healthcare professionals from the Centers for Disease Control and Prevention and the American Heart Association. Circulation. 2003;107(3):499–511.
39. Ridker PM, Rifai N, Clearfield M, Downs JR, Weis SE, Miles JS, et al. Measurement of C-reactive protein for the targeting of statin therapy in the primary prevention of acute coronary events. N Engl J Med. 2001;344(26):1959–65.
40. Ridker PM, Cannon CP, Morrow D, Rifai N, Rose LM, McCabe CH, et al. C-reactive protein levels and outcomes after statin therapy. N Engl J Med. 2005;352(1):20–8.
41. Braunwald E. Creating controversy where none exists: the important role of C-reactive protein in the CARE, AFCAPS/TexCAPS, PROVE IT, REVERSAL, A to Z, JUPITER, HEART PROTECTION, and ASCOT trials. Eur Heart J. 2012;33(4):430–2.
42. Ridker PM, Danielson E, Fonseca FA, Genest J, Gotto Jr AM, Kastelein JJ, et al. Rosuvastatin to prevent vascular events in men and women with elevated C-reactive protein. N Engl J Med. 2008;359(21):2195–207.
43. Mora S, Glynn RJ, Hsia J, Macfadyen JG, Genest J, Ridker PM. Statins for the primary prevention of cardiovascular events in women with elevated high-sensitivity C-reactive protein or dyslipidemia. Results from the Justification for the Use of Statins in Prevention: An intervention trial evaluating rosuvastatin (JUPITER) and meta-analysis of women from primary prevention trials. Circulation. 2010;121(9):1069–77.
44. Glynn RJ, Koenig W, Nordestgaard BG, Shepherd J, Ridker PM. Rosuvastatin for primary prevention in older persons with elevated C-reactive protein and low to average low-density lipoprotein cholesterol levels: exploratory analysis of a randomized trial. Ann Intern Med. 2010;152(8):488–96.
45. Ridker PM. Moving beyond JUPITER: will inhibiting inflammation reduce vascular event rates? Curr Atheroscler Rep. 2013;15(1):295.
46. Ridker PM, MacFadyen JG, Fonseca FA, Genest J, Gotto AM, Kastelein JJ, et al. Number needed to treat with rosuvastatin to prevent first cardiovascular events and death among men and women with low low-density lipoprotein cholesterol and elevated high-sensitivity C-reactive protein: justification for the use of statins in prevention: an intervention trial evaluating rosuvastatin (JUPITER). Circ Cardiovasc Qual Outcomes. 2009;2(6):616–23.
47. Ridker PM, Thuren T, Zalewski A, Libby P. Interleukin-1beta inhibition and the prevention of recurrent cardiovascular events: rationale and design of the Canakinumab Anti-inflammatory Thrombosis Outcomes Study (CANTOS). Am Heart J. 2011;162(4):597–605.
48. Ridker PM. Testing the inflammatory hypothesis of atherothrombosis: scientific rationale for the cardiovascular inflammation reduction trial (CIRT). J Thromb Haemost. 2009;7 Suppl 1:332–9.
49. Koenig W. Fibrinogen in cardiovascular disease: an update. Thromb Haemost. 2003;89(4):601–9.
50. Ridker PM, Stampfer MJ, Rifai N. Novel risk factors for systemic atherosclerosis: a comparison of C-reactive protein, fibrinogen, homocysteine, lipoprotein(a), and standard cholesterol screening as predictors of peripheral arterial disease. JAMA. 2001;285(19):2481–5.

51. Artl A, Marsche G, Lestavel S, Sattler W, Malle E. Role of serum amyloid A during metabolism of acute-phase HDL by macrophages. Arterioscler Thromb Vasc Biol. 2000;20(3):763–72.
52. Morrow DA, Rifai N, Antman EM, Weiner DL, McCabe CH, Cannon CP, et al. Serum amyloid A predicts early mortality in acute coronary syndromes: a TIMI 11A substudy. J Am Coll Cardiol. 2000;35(2):358–62.
53. Tedgui A, Mallat Z. Cytokines in atherosclerosis: pathogenic and regulatory pathways. Physiol Rev. 2006;86(2):515–81.
54. McKellar GE, McCarey DW, Sattar N, McInnes IB. Role for TNF in atherosclerosis? Lessons from autoimmune disease. Nat Rev Cardiol. 2009;6(6):410–7.
55. Nieto-Vazquez I, Fernández-Veledo S, Krämer DK, Vila-Bedmar R, Garcia-Guerra L, Lorenzo M. Insulin resistance associated to obesity: the link TNF-alpha. Arch Physiol Biochem. 2008;114(3):183–94.
56. Ridker PM, Rifai N, Pfeffer M, Sacks F, Lepage S, Braunwald E. Elevation of tumor necrosis factor-alpha and increased risk of recurrent coronary events after myocardial infarction. Circulation. 2000;101(18):2149–53.
57. Schuett H, Luchtefeld M, Grothusen C, Grote K, Schieffer B. How much is too much? Interleukin-6 and its signalling in atherosclerosis. Thromb Haemost. 2009;102(2):215–22.
58. Ridker PM, Rifai N, Stampfer MJ, Hennekens CH. Plasma concentration of interleukin-6 and the risk of future myocardial infarction among apparently healthy men. Circulation. 2000;101(15):1767–72.
59. Lutgens E, Lievens D, Beckers L, Donners M, Daemen M. CD40 and its ligand in atherosclerosis. Trends Cardiovasc Med. 2007;17(4):118–23.
60. Heeschen C, Dimmeler S, Hamm CW, van den Brand MJ, Boersma E, Zeiher AM, et al. Soluble CD40 ligand in acute coronary syndromes. N Engl J Med. 2003;348(12):1104–11.
61. Heeschen C, Dimmeler S, Hamm CW, Fichtlscherer S, Boersma E, Simoons ML, et al. Serum level of the antiinflammatory cytokine interleukin-10 is an important prognostic determinant in patients with acute coronary syndromes. Circulation. 2003;107(16):2109–14.
62. Jha HC, Divya A, Prasad J, Mittal A. Plasma circulatory markers in male and female patients with coronary artery disease. Heart Lung. 2010;39(4):296–303.
63. Cipollone F, Fazia M, Mincione G, Iezzi A, Pini B, Cuccurullo C, et al. Increased expression of transforming growth factor-β1 as a stabilizing factor in human atherosclerotic plaques. Stroke. 2004;35:2253–7.
64. Stefoni S, Cianciolo G, Donati G, Dormi A, Silvestri MG, Colì L, et al. Low TGF-β1 serum levels are a risk factor for atherosclerosis disease in ESRD patients. Kidney Int. 2002;61:324–35.
65. Koch W, Hoppmann P, Mueller JC, Schomig A, Kastrati A. Association of transforming growth factor-β1 gene polymorphisms with myocardial infarction in patients with angiographically proven coronary heart disease. Arterioscler Thromb Vasc Biol. 2006;26:1114–9.
66. Ouchi N, Shibata R, Walsh K. Cardioprotection by adiponectin. Trends Cardiovasc Med. 2006;16(5):141–6.
67. Pischon T, Girman CJ, Hotamisligil GS, Rifai N, Hu FB, Rimm EB. Plasma adiponectin levels and risk of myocardial infarction in men. JAMA. 2004;291(14):1730–7.
68. Frystyk J, Berne C, Berglund L, Jensevik K, Flyvbjerg A, Zethelius B. Serum adiponectin is a predictor of coronary heart disease: a population-based 10-year follow-up study in elderly men. J Clin Endocrinol Metab. 2007;92(2):571–6.
69. Miwa K, Igawa A, Inoue H. Soluble E-selectin, ICAM-1 and VCAM-1 levels in systemic and coronary circulation in patients with variant angina. Cardiovasc Res. 1997;36(1):37–44.
70. Roldan V, Marin F, Lip GY, Blann AD. Soluble E-selectin in cardiovascular disease and its risk factors. A review of the literature. Thromb Haemost. 2003;90(6):1007–20.
71. Luc G, Arveiler D, Evans A, Amouyel P, Ferrieres J, Bard JM, et al. Circulating soluble adhesion molecules ICAM-1 and VCAM-1 and incident coronary heart disease: the PRIME Study. Atherosclerosis. 2003;170(1):169–76.

72. Jenny NS, Arnold AM, Kuller LH, Sharrett AR, Fried LP, Psaty BM, et al. Soluble intercellular adhesion molecule-1 is associated with cardiovascular disease risk and mortality in older adults. J Thromb Haemost. 2006;4(1):107–13.
73. Blankenberg S, Rupprecht HJ, Bickel C, Peetz D, Hafner G, Tiret L, et al. Circulating cell adhesion molecules and death in patients with coronary artery disease. Circulation. 2001;104(12):1336–42.
74. Braunersreuther V, Mach F, Steffens S. The specific role of chemokines in atherosclerosis. Thromb Haemost. 2007;97(5):714–21.
75. Prondzinsky R, Unverzagt S, Lemm H, Wegener NA, Schlitt A, Heinroth KM, et al. Interleukin-6, −7, −8 and −10 predict outcome in acute myocardial infarction complicated by cardiogenic shock. Clin Res Cardiol. 2012;101:375–84.
76. Burger-Kentischer A, Goebel H, Seiler R, Fraedrich G, Schaefer HE, Dimmeler S, et al. Expression of macrophage migration inhibitory factor in different stages of human atherosclerosis. Circulation. 2002;105(13):1561–6.
77. Herder C, Illig T, Baumert J, Muller M, Klopp N, Khuseyinova N, et al. Macrophage migration inhibitory factor (MIF) and risk for coronary heart disease: results from the MONICA/KORA Augsburg case-cohort study, 1984–2002. Atherosclerosis. 2008;200(2):380–8.
78. Martinovic I, Abegunewardene N, Seul M, Vosseler M, Horstick G, Buerke M, et al. Elevated monocyte chemoattractant protein-1 serum levels in patients at risk for coronary artery disease. Circ J. 2005;69(12):1484–9.
79. Lijnen HR. Plasmin and matrix metalloproteinases in vascular remodeling. Thromb Haemost. 2001;86(1):324–33.
80. Inokubo Y, Hanada H, Ishizaka H, Fukushi T, Kamada T, Okumura K. Plasma levels of matrix metalloproteinase-9 and tissue inhibitor of metalloproteinase-1 are increased in the coronary circulation in patients with acute coronary syndrome. Am Heart J. 2001;141:211–7.
81. Nicholls SJ, Hazen SL. Myeloperoxidase and cardiovascular disease. Arterioscler Thromb Vasc Biol. 2005;25:1102–11.
82. Vita JA, Brennan M-L, Gokce N, Mann SA, Goormastic M, Shishehbor MH, et al. Serum myeloperoxidase levels independently predict endothelial dysfunction in humans. Circulation. 2004;110(9):1134–9.
83. Baldus S, Heeschen C, Meinertz T, Zeiher AM, Eiserich JP, Munzel T, et al. Myeloperoxidase serum levels predict risk in patients with acute coronary syndromes. Circulation. 2003;108(12):1440–5.

Chapter 2
Cardiovascular Disease

Andreia Fernandes, Rui Providência, Flávio Reis, and Lino Gonçalves

Abstract Inflammatory mechanisms play a major role in the pathogenesis of vascular and cardiac diseases. Several immune cells (including macrophages and T cells) participate in all stages of atherosclerosis, including initiation, progression, and plaque destabilization and rupture. Inflammation seems to play also a significant role in the beginning, maintenance, and perpetuation of atrial fibrillation (AF), the most common arrhythmia in clinical practice. It is not clear yet if inflammation occurs as a cause or a consequence of AF, but several inflammatory markers are elevated in AF and correlate to the outcomes of different rhythm control strategies and thrombogenesis.

Keywords Cardiovascular disease • Inflammation • Inflammatory cells • Atherosclerosis • Atrial fibrillation • Biomarkers • C-reactive protein

Introduction

The concept of cardiovascular disease (CVD) refers to a class of diseases that affect the heart, the blood vessels, or both and includes clinical entities such as myocardial infarction (MI), atrial fibrillation (AF), valvular heart disease, coronary heart disease (CHD), coronary artery disease (CAD), peripheral arterial disease, heart failure, stroke, and claudication, among others. CVD is the main cause of death in the Western world, and, according to the World Health Organization, its prevalence is expected to increase. In fact, CVD is responsible for almost 40 % of all deaths in

A. Fernandes, M.D. • R. Providência, M.D., M.Sc. • L. Gonçalves, M.D., Ph.D. (✉)
Department of Cardiology – B, Centro Hospitalar e Universitário de Coimbra,
Quinta dos Vales, S. Martinho do Bispo, Coimbra 3041-801, Portugal
e-mail: lgoncalv@ci.uc.pt

F. Reis, Ph.D.
Laboratory of Pharmacology and Experimental Therapeutics, Institute for Biomedical Imaging and Life Sciences (IBILI), and CNC.IBILI Research Unit, Faculty of Medicine, Coimbra University, Coimbra, Portugal

© Springer International Publishing Switzerland 2015

F. Palavra et al. (eds.), *Biomarkers of Cardiometabolic Risk, Inflammation and Disease*, DOI 10.1007/978-3-319-16018-4_2

North America and in Europe; it is the main cause of premature death in women, being responsible for 42 % of all deaths below 75 years of age in European women and for 38 % of all deaths in men less than 75 years old [1].

Atherosclerosis is the underlying cause of most cardiovascular diseases. Although the central event is the development of atherosclerotic plaques in the inner lining of arteries, the pathophysiology of the disease is complex and multifactorial, involving accumulation of modified lipids and foam cells in a necrotic core, with participation of several other cells, including vascular endothelial and smooth muscle cells, progenitor cells, and platelets, as well as inflammatory cells, including monocyte-derived macrophages, T lymphocytes, and vascular dendritic cells. This complexity and the diversity of risk factors involved, some of them non-modifiable, might explain the failure to eliminate or at least to seriously reduce to residual levels the consequences of atherosclerosis. Despite the remarkable impact obtained using lipid-lowering therapy, namely, statins, the epidemiological data remain alarming, and there is a "residual" cardiovascular risk, even after aggressive statin therapy that deserves renewed efforts and more efficient answers. The traditional risk algorithms, such as the Framingham risk score (FRS), which includes risk factors such as age, male sex, hypercholesterolemia, arterial hypertension, and smoking, seem to be unable to identify patients' residual cardiovascular risk, and new/better risk factors/markers are needed to improve risk prediction and prognosis as well as to monitor therapeutics' efficacy.

Inflammatory mechanisms play a central role in all phases of atherosclerosis, from lesion initiation to progression and destabilization/rupture of the unstable plaque [2, 3]. Thus, great attention has been focused on whether risk factors and/or biomarkers of inflammation could be pivotal in identifying those patients at high risk for future cardiovascular events, as well as to dissect the effectiveness of therapeutic agents. The clinical utility of new molecules (whether risk factors and/or markers) cannot be estimated before a profound knowledge on the role played by inflammation (and by mediators of inflammation) in the pathogenic processes of atherogenesis and plaque destabilization. That is, even though it is now widely recognized and accepted that atherosclerosis is an inflammatory disease, the precise identification and characterization of the players of this process, the regulatory mechanisms, and the specific pathogenic consequences remain to be elucidated.

Atrial fibrillation (AF) is the most common cardiac arrhythmia with a prevalence of 1.5–2 % in the general population [4]. The prevalence of AF doubles with each advancing decade after the age of 50 [5, 6]. Considering the advancing age of the population, thousands of millions of subjects will suffer from AF and its consequences in the next decades [7]. This arrhythmia is more common in patients with a history of cardiovascular disease and is associated with increased morbidity, mortality, and financial costs, as well as with a fivefold risk of stroke and a higher risk of developing heart failure [8–12]. Despite the extensive studies, pathophysiological mechanisms in AF remain partially unclear. Inflammation has been associated with numerous cardiovascular diseases such as hypertension, atherosclerosis, and metabolic syndrome [13, 14]. Recently, researchers have started to focus on the role of inflammation in the pathogenesis of AF.

This chapter focuses on the interplay between inflammation and cardiovascular diseases. In particular, authors will dissect the involvement of inflammatory mechanisms in the different phases of atherosclerotic lesion, as the prototype model of vascular disease, including the role played, and the putative biomarkers associated with initiation, lesion progression, and plaque destabilization and rupture. Additionally, the relationship between inflammation and AF will be analyzed, as an example of a cardiac disease, focusing on the involvement of inflammatory mechanisms, and possible biomarkers, in AF genesis, perpetuation, and thromboembolic complications. Lastly, the possible therapeutic options will be discussed.

Participation of Inflammatory Mechanisms in Atherosclerotic Lesion

Recruitment of Inflammatory Cells to the Artery Wall in the Initiation Phase

Atherosclerosis was long viewed essentially as a lipid disorder starting with accumulation of modified lipids in the artery wall. Advances in vascular biology have clearly established the involvement of the innate immune system in the disease, and nowadays it is recognized that both lipid modification and accumulation and inflammatory mechanisms are pivotal in the initiation and evolution of the disease [15]. Figures 2.1 and 2.2 schematically summarize the inflammatory mechanisms participating in all stages of atherosclerosis lesion development, from initiation, progression, and destabilization and rupture.

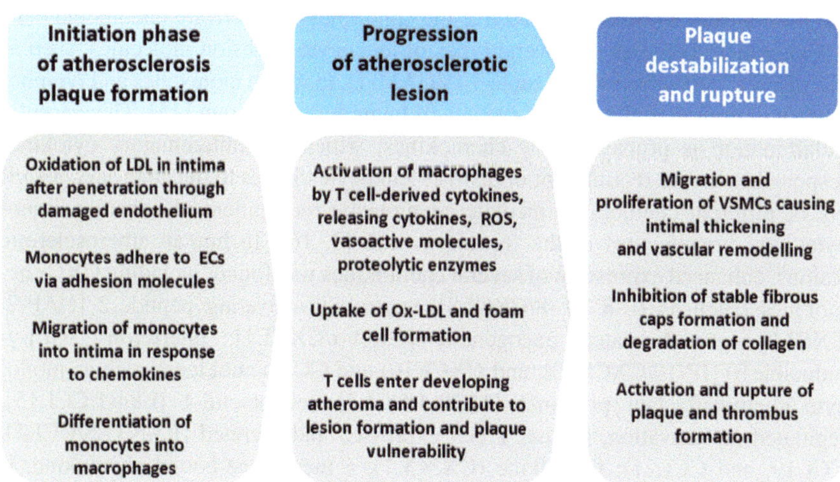

Fig. 2.1 Main inflammatory mechanisms participating in atherosclerotic lesion initiation, progression, and plaque destabilization and rupture

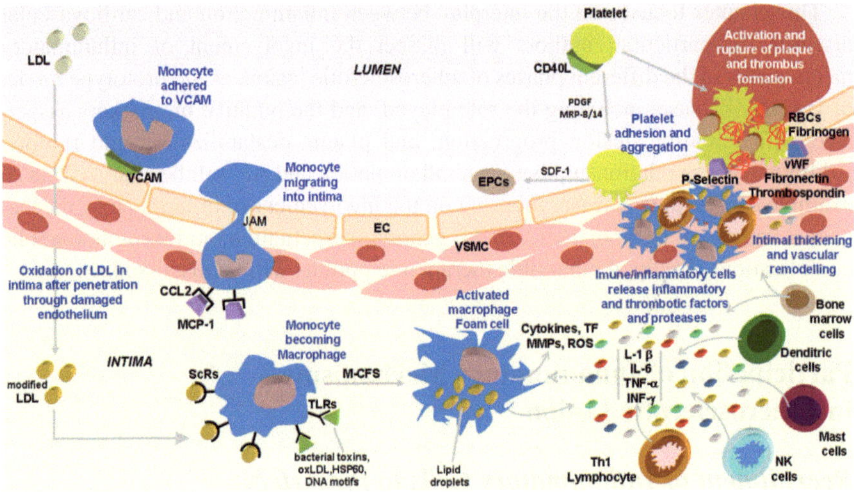

Fig. 2.2 Vascular and immune inflammatory cells that participate in atherosclerosis and main molecular mediators involved in atherosclerotic lesion initiation, progression, and plaque destabilization and rupture

It has been suggested that the early phase of atherosclerosis is better explained as an inflammatory response caused by retention of lipoproteins in the arterial intima. The increased amount of cholesterol-rich very low-density lipoprotein (VLDL) and low-density lipoprotein (LDL) in circulation, and the existence of a damaged endothelium, elicits lipoprotein infiltration in the artery wall and accumulation in the extracellular matrix. This accumulation exceeds the capacity for elimination, and this is the initiating pathological process of atherosclerosis [2]. LDL oxidation in the intima causes release of bioactive phospholipids that activate endothelial cells (ECs), which then express several types of leukocyte adhesion molecules, such as the vascular cell adhesion molecule-1 (VCAM-1), to which monocytes and lymphocytes will preferentially adhere, at sites of hemodynamic strain [15]. This vascular inflammation is propagated by chemokines, which are inflammatory cytokines responsible for the recruitment of distinct leukocyte classes to the atheroma; a variety of different chemokines mediate chemotactic recruitment of adherent monocytes and lymphocytes to the forming lesion [3, 16]. In human atherosclerotic lesions, enhanced expression of several chemokines was found, including CXC chemokines (such as IL-8 [IL-8/CXCL8], neutrophil-activating peptide-2 [NAP-2/CXCL7], growth-related oncogene-α [GRO-α/CXCL1], interferon [INF]-γ-inducible10 [IP-10/CXCL10], and CXCL16) and CC chemokines (such as monocyte chemoattractant protein-1 [MCP-1/CCL2], leukotactin-1 [Lkn-1/CCL15], regulated on activation, normal T cell expressed and secreted [RANTES/CCL5], CCL19, and CCL21); fractalkine (CX3CL1), a membrane-bound chemokine, is also expressed and promotes recruitment of CX3CR1+ mononuclear cells to the lesion area.

Transmigration of monocytes occurs mainly in areas where the basal lamina is enriched with modified LDL and via endothelial cell junctions (junction adhesion molecule [JAM]-A and [JAM]-C), which are implicated in the control of vascular permeability and leukocyte transmigration (Fig. 2.2) [17]. Chemokines have been viewed as the link between lipidic and inflammatory pathways in atherogenesis, which is supported by the fact that modified LDL particles elicit chemokine stimulation in macrophages and vascular smooth muscle cells (VSMCs), among other cells [3, 16].

Chemoattractant factors, which include monocyte chemoattractant protein-1 (MCP-1 or CCL2) produced by vascular wall cells in response to modified lipoproteins, are responsible for the migration and diapedesis of adherent monocytes [16]. Monocytic cells directly interacting with human ECs increase severalfold the production of monocyte matrix metalloproteinase 9 (MMP-9), leading to subsequent infiltration of leukocytes through the endothelial layer [18]. The inflamed intima produces the macrophage colony-stimulating factor (M-CSF), a cytokine/growth factor that is responsible for the differentiation of monocytes into macrophages [15]. This process is associated with macrophage overexpression of pattern recognition receptors for innate immunity, including scavenger receptors (ScRs) and Toll-like receptors (TLRs) (Fig. 2.2) [19]. ScRs use receptor-mediated endocytosis to engulf and degrade a broad range of molecules and particles carrying pathogen-like molecular patterns, including oxidized lipoproteins (in particular, oxidized LDL [oxLDL]), bacterial endotoxins, and apoptotic cell fragments. Accumulation of cholesterol esters in the cytoplasm droplets, aggravated by pro-inflammatory cytokines and endotoxins that inhibit the expression of ATP-binding cassette transporters ABCA1 and ABCG1 responsible for cholesterol efflux from the cell, converts macrophages into foam cells, which are lipid-laden macrophages typical of early-stage atherosclerosis. On the other hand, and unlike ScRs, TLRs do not mediate endocytosis, but bind ligands with pathogen-like molecular patterns (such as bacterial toxins, oxLDL, stress proteins such as heat shock protein 60 [HSP60], and DNA motifs), initiating a cascade that culminates in macrophage activation [19]. This process also occurs in dendritic cells, mast cells, and endothelial cells, all of them possessing TLRs (Fig. 2.2).

Additional mechanisms contribute to the inflammatory milieu within the lesion that determines plaque formation, including advanced glycation end products (AGE) that, after binding to receptors for AGE (RAGE) on macrophages, ECs, and VSMCs, causes amplification of vascular inflammation due to activation of nuclear factor kappa B (NF-κB). Moreover, activated macrophage produces reactive oxygen species (ROS) and triggers the release of vasoactive molecules, including endothelins, eicosanoids, and nitric oxide, altogether contributing to amplify lipoprotein oxidation and cytotoxicity [15]. These macrophages also secrete proteolytic enzymes that are able to degrade matrix components, thus having a later role on destabilization of plaques and contributing to an increased risk for plaque rupture and thrombosis (Figs. 2.1 and 2.2).

Role of Inflammatory Mediators in Atherosclerotic Lesion Progression

Whereas foam cell accumulation characterizes fatty streaks, deposition of fibrous tissue defines the more advanced atherosclerotic lesion [20]. Macrophage-derived foam cells are crucial in lesion progression because they amplify the inflammatory response through the secretion of numerous growth factors and cytokines, including tumor necrosis factor-α (TNF-α) and interleukin (IL)-1β (Fig. 2.2). In addition, T lymphocytes join macrophages in the intima and govern the adaptive immune responses. These cells, as well as ECs, secrete additional cytokines and growth factors that promote the migration and proliferation of VSMCs (Fig. 2.2). In response to inflammatory stimulation, VSMCs express specialized enzymes that can degrade elastin and collagen, allowing their penetration into the expanding lesion.

Chemokines within the plaque elicit activation of ECs and different leukocyte subsets (such as T cells), causing additional release of inflammatory cytokines and chemokines, which then promote further recruitment and activation of leukocytes, in a cycle of amplification of inflammation [3, 16]. Chemokine receptor CXCR3 interacts with its ligands (CXCL9 [MIG], CXCL10 [IP-10], and CXCL11 [I-TAC]) and promotes an inflammatory T-cell phenotype that causes macrophage activation [16]. Activation of macrophages also occurs directly by chemokines, which trigger increased release of cytokines and production of tissue factor (TF), MMPs, and ROS, and enhanced lipid loading and foam cell formation by upregulation of scavenger receptors. Altogether, these mechanisms, and the interaction between MCP-1 and CCR2, will highly alter macrophages to a pro-inflammatory, matrix-degrading, procoagulant, and proapoptotic phenotype [16].

Beyond their effects on T cells and macrophages, chemokines also interfere with VSMCs. While chemokines may promote VSMC migration into the lesion, an early event in atherogenesis, they could also transform these cells from a nonproliferative contractile phenotype, typical in healthy arteries, into actively proliferative cells (synthetic phenotype), which migrate when attracted by chemotactic agents, and increase matrix synthesis [16]. The migration of VSMCs from the vascular media to the intima is a hallmark process in intimal thickening and vascular remodeling characterizing atherosclerosis (Fig. 2.1). Recent data suggests that circulating bone marrow cells and progenitor cells present in the adventitia may also be a potential source of VSMCs in the intima [21] (Fig. 2.2).

T lymphocytes have been shown to contribute to atherogenesis and lesion development and progression [22, 23]. T cells are recruited to the forming lesion by mechanisms similar to those described for monocytes, despite using different patterns of activation, which is dependent upon recognition of cognate antigens and concomitant ligation of costimulatory receptors. Adhesion molecules (such as VCAM-1) and chemokines trigger T cells to enter the atheroma, where they react to several local molecules (peptide antigens) bound to major histocompatibility complex (MHC) molecules on the surface of antigen-presenting cells (APCs), such as oxLDL, HSP60, and microbial antigens. T-cell activation elicits distinct responses, involving T-helper-1 (Th1) cells, regulatory T cells (Treg), Th2 cells, and natural killer (NK) T cells [15, 22]. The precise role played by Th2 cells remains to be elucidated, while NK T cells recognize lipid antigens presented by CD1 molecules and trigger responses identical to those elicited by MHC-restricted T cells, including release of pro-inflammatory mediators and progression of lesion. While Th1 response, the most common in atheroma, involves induction of pro-inflammatory cytokines and promotion of lesion formation, Treg cells have an inhibitory effect on this process. In fact, Th1 cells produce IFN-γ, TNF-α, and CD40 ligand (CD40L), among other mediators, which are responsible for several responses. IFN-γ elicits activation of macrophages and endothelial cells via production of adhesion molecules, cytokines, chemokines, radicals, proteases, and coagulation factors, thus contributing to atherogenic lesion progression. TNF-α is produced by Th1 cells, but also by macrophages and NK cells, and has pro-inflammatory effects via NF-κB pathways [15, 22]. Other cytokines also play important roles in the atherogenic process [3, 16]. IL-18 receptor is expressed in endothelial and VSMCs, as well as in macrophages, and this cytokine elicits several important actions in atherogenesis, including induction of adhesion molecules (namely, VCAM-1), chemokines (i.e., IL-8), cytokines (in particular, IL-6), and several [1, 9, 13] MPPs, and, in combination with IL-12, upregulates the expression of IFN-γ in T cells, in macrophages, and in VSMCs, thus influencing important pro-inflammatory pathways involved in atherogenesis [16]. In opposition to Th1 cells, Treg cells are implicated in the maintenance of self-tolerance and regulation of autoimmunity, and the anti-inflammatory properties seem to derive from the production of transforming growth factor beta (TGF-β) and/or IL-10. T cells in atheroma display an activated/memory phenotype, and the proportion of activated T cells is particularly high in advanced lesions causing acute coronary syndrome (ACS).

The contribution of vascular dendritic cells (DCs) and mast cells to atherogenesis progression has been also suggested [24]. Although the exact role of vascular DCs remains poorly understood, they are thought to show antigen to naïve T cells accelerating lymphocyte recruitment into the atherosclerotic vessel. Mast cells seem to coordinate both the innate and acquired immunity through the activation of TLRs and cytokine release (Fig. 2.2).

Platelets also play a major role in the pathogenesis of atherosclerosis by several mechanisms, including production of inflammatory mediators (such as CD40L, myeloid-related protein-8/14 [MRP-8/14], and platelet-derived growth factor [PDGF]), and elicit leukocyte adhesion and incorporation into plaques, which is a robust example of the interplay between inflammation and thrombosis in the biology of atherothrombosis (Fig. 2.2) [20]. Platelets, as well as other cells involved in the disease (ECs and VSMCs, macrophages, and T cells), express CD40L and its receptor CD40 [25]. This pro-inflammatory cytokine plays a relevant role in this stage of atherogenesis, including stimulation of expression of adhesion molecules and of secretion of cytokines and MMPs which are involved in the degradation of extracellular matrix, as well as expression of tissue factor in ECs, VSMCs, and macrophages, which is responsible for the initiation of the coagulation cascade when exposed to factor VII. Thus,

CD40L participates in the molecular events that will contribute to destabilization of plaques and increases the risk for plaque rupture and thrombosis.

Inflammatory Activation and Rupture of Plaque

Plaque rupture and the ensuing thrombosis commonly cause the most serious acute complications of atherosclerosis. Recent data suggest that inflammatory mechanisms, including infiltration and activation of leukocytes into the atherosclerotic plaque, rather than the degree of stenosis, are involved in plaque destabilization and rupture, resulting in coronary thrombosis leading to myocardial ischemia and infarction, for example (Fig. 2.1). In fact, ACS patients present typical features of an inflammatory phenotype, presenting several blood disturbances including increased contents of acute-phase reactants, cytokines, and activated T cells.

Plaque destabilization seems to occur due to the action of several types of molecules, including pro-inflammatory cytokines, chemokines, proteases, coagulation factors, vasoactive molecules, and radicals, mainly produced by activated macrophages, T cells, and mast cells located at sites of rupture (Fig. 2.2) [15, 16, 20]. These mediators are involved in several mechanisms that promote plaque activation, rupture, thrombosis, and ischemia, including inhibition of stable fibrous cap formation, degradation of collagen cap, and initiation of thrombus formation. Chemokines have been associated with the immune-mediated plaque destabilization due to several distinct mechanisms, namely, recruiting of activated leukocytes, stimulation of matrix degradation by macrophages, and induction of tissue factor in vascular ECs and VSMCs, as well as by promotion of oxidative stress and apoptosis in the plaques [16]. In addition, besides their role in thrombus formation, platelets could also have a major role on ACS, namely, due to release of pro-inflammatory mediators, including chemokines (such as CCL5, CXCL1, CXCL7, and epithelial neutrophil-activating peptide-78 [ENA-78/CXCL5]), and due to exacerbated inflammation in leukocytes and ECs [16].

The inflammatory milieu within atherosclerotic plaques stimulates the degradation of collagen fibers and inhibits the formation of new collagen, thus impairing the integrity of the interstitial collagen of the fibrous cap. In addition, activated T cells secrete IFN-γ which inhibits production of collagen by VSMCs. T lymphocytes are involved in several mechanisms that contribute to plaque destabilization, including production of IL-1 and CD40L which elicits macrophages to release interstitial collagenases, including MMPs [1, 8, 9, 13], that were detected in the shoulder region of plaques as well as in areas of foam cell accumulation, where activation and rupture of the plaque occur [22, 23]. MMPs are involved in the deregulation of extracellular matrix and intravascular thrombus formation, due to overexpression of tissue factor and activation of the coagulation cascade, thus contributing to plaque rupture [26].

Proteolytic destruction of collagen and inhibition of VSMC growth cause the reduction of cap thickness and strength, which become unable to support the hemodynamic forces and fissures, thus exposing components of the vascular matrix, including, e.g., different types of collagen, von Willebrand factor (vWF), fibronectin, laminin, fibulin, and thrombospondin (Fig. 2.2) [24]. ACS widely occurs due to physical disruption of the fibrous cap, either frank cap fracture or superficial endothelial erosion. The contact of blood with thrombogenic material (platelets and coagulation factors) initiates the formation of a thrombus, which can lead to abrupt and impressive obstruction of blood flow through the affected artery, and ischemia occurs in the end organ, such as the myocardium or the brain [20]. When the thrombus is nonocclusive or transient, the result could be clinically silent or cause symptoms typical of an ACS, including acute MI, unstable angina, or sudden death. The concentrations of circulating plasminogen activator inhibitor 1 (PAI-1) and fibrinogen usually determine the fate of a given plaque disruption [20].

Inflammatory Mediators as Biomarkers in Cardiovascular Disease

Considering the role played by inflammation in all the stages of atherosclerotic disease, a variety of inflammatory mediators have been tested, in experimental and in clinical studies, as putative biomarkers of the pathogenic mechanisms that underlie the initiation and evolution of the disease, as well as predictors of risk and future events. The main question is whether plasma markers of inflammation can be noninvasively and feasibly used to improve diagnosis and prognosis of distinct forms of atherosclerosis.

The putative biomarkers of inflammation include different types of molecules, such as acute-phase reactants (namely, C-reactive protein [CRP], serum amyloid A (SAA) proteins, and fibrinogen), cytokines (including IL-1β, TNF-α, IL-6, and IFN-γ), adipokines (i.e., adiponectin), adhesion molecules (such as selectins and VCAM-1), platelet products (namely, CD40 ligand and MRP-8/14), and proteases (namely, MMP-9) [15, 16, 20]. Some of these analytes may participate in a pathogenic pathway, but not acting as an effective biomarker, while others may reflect the local inflammatory process in the artery, but do not have a causal role on the disease (thus acting as a biomarker, but not as a risk factor).

CRP has been viewed as the prototype of inflammatory markers. Accumulated evidence suggests that it could be a feasible marker of cardiovascular risk in MI patients, which presents augmented levels, and a predictor of future events in apparently healthy individuals [27, 28]. The development of a high-sensitivity assay for CRP (hsCRP) allowed accurate measurement of this molecule as a tool to enhance risk stratification. In fact, hsCRP has been shown predictive value beyond that of traditional risk factors, at least in specific populations with intermediate risk according to conventional criteria (namely, the Framingham algorithm), to whom the determination of hsCRP was already suggested (by US Centers for Disease Control and Prevention [CDC] and American Heart Association [AHA]) as a way to improve identification and stratification of risk [29]. Note that this intermediate risk group accounts for much of the burden of cardiovascular events recommending improved prediction tools. The Reynolds risk score adds hsCRP (as well as the family history of premature CAD) to traditional risk factors in a clinically useful manner [30].

Considering a successful application to identify and stratify cardiovascular risk, as well as its independence from traditional risk factors (namely, hypercholesterolemia), biomarkers of inflammation were suggested as a way to identify individuals who might benefit from therapeutic intervention, regardless of low estimates of cardiovascular risk according on traditional risk factors. The JUPITER (*Justification for the Use of Statins in Prevention: an Intervention Trial Evaluating Rosuvastatin*) trial enrolled more than 17,000 individuals without known CVD, low LDL-c levels (<130 mg/dL), and hsCRP >2 mg/L in order to evaluate the effect of statin therapy in cardiovascular events and mortality [31, 32]. The results showed a major (>40 %) reduction of events and all-cause mortality, and additional analyses suggested that the benefits could be derived both from LDL reduction and improved anti-inflammatory effect viewed by hsCRP reduction. Evidence that a direct anti-inflammatory therapy positively impacts on atherosclerotic events cannot be drawn from the study, but ongoing trials (*Canakinumab Anti-Inflammatory Thrombosis Outcomes Study* [CANTOS] and *Cardiovascular Inflammation Reduction Trial* [CIRT]) could provide evidence on this, which is expected to have a major impact in the way CVD could be managed in the near future.

All these putative useful roles played by hsCRP need to be precisely defined through adequate and larger clinical trials that may test a number of targets and mediators. At the moment, doubts remain whether CRP could alone reflect the inflammatory mechanisms underlying atherosclerosis development, especially knowing the involvement of several other mediators (including a variety of cytokines), whether CRP could be viewed as a risk factor (with a causal role) or just as a surrogate marker of the process, and finally whether CRP or any other emergent biomarker of inflammation and cardiovascular risk could effectively and consistently improve clinical performance (namely, diagnosis, prediction of risk and/or of mortality, therapeutic decisions) in distinct populations.

The validation of the concept that inflammation is crucial for atherogenesis and its translation to clinical practice is an ongoing mission that deserves continuous efforts.

Inflammatory Mechanisms Involved in Atrial Fibrillation

Pathophysiology of Atrial Fibrillation

The development of abnormal tissue substrate allows multiple reentrant wavelets of excitation to propagate within the atrial myocardium contributing for the maintenance of AF [33]. As AF episodes get more frequent and/or prolonged, restoring and maintaining sinus rhythm becomes more difficult – "*AF begets AF*" [34]. This is the result of electrical remodeling and electrophysiological changes such as shortening of the atrial effective refractory period and action potential duration [33]. During structural remodeling, myocyte degeneration and myocardial fibrosis occur, leading to left atrial enlargement [34]. These changes create a susceptible substrate that has been implicated in the perpetuation of AF.

Garrey in 1914 proposed the "critical mass theory" of fibrillation. This hypothesis went nearly unchallenged for over 60 years and was based on the fact that multiple, changing reentrant circuits, modified by refractory tissue areas, caused the irregular activity seen during AF [35]. According to this theory, there is a critical mass above which AF is sustained, meaning that the greater the atrial tissue surface area, the higher the probability of having sustained episodes of arrhythmia [35]. This mass is correlated with the area of geometric/structural and functional abnormalities. However, almost 20 years ago, Haïssaguere and colleagues in a seminal investigation identified pulmonary veins as the initiators of AF episodes and first assessed radiofrequency ablation as an effective way of treating this arrhythmia [36].

Inflammation is associated with electrophysiological and structural atrial remodeling and facilitates the disease development and perpetuation [33]. Several histological findings confirming the presence of active inflammation in patients with AF are known to occur. Nakamura et al. found active atrial perimyocarditis with inflammatory infiltrates, lipid degeneration, and fibrosis in patients with nonvalvular AF and cardiogenic thromboembolism [37]. Frustaci et al. have shown in atrial biopsies from patients with AF a higher prevalence of inflammatory infiltrates, myocyte necrosis, and fibrosis, whereas biopsies from control subjects were normal [38]. More recently, Narducci et al. assessed atrial inflammation by the identification of CRP in atrial cardiomyocytes. CRP was more frequent in paroxysmal rather than in persistent AF patients and wasn't present in the control group [39].

The possible association between AF and inflammation is suggested by several studies based on the identification of inflammatory serum biomarkers that are elevated in patients with AF. Considering the existent published data, inflammation may be linked with the initiation and perpetuation of AF and also with the increased thrombotic burden of this population [40].

Inflammatory Markers in Atrial Fibrillation

Table 2.1 presents the main studies involving inflammatory markers and atrial fibrillation.

C-Reactive Protein and the Development of Atrial Fibrillation

CRP is a marker of the magnitude of inflammation and is widely used in the clinical setting [41]. It has been used to detect acute injury, infection, and inflammation [41, 48]. It is an acute-phase protein produced in the liver in response to IL-1, IL-6, and TNF-α that binds to damaged cells, activating the complement pathway [41].

Table 2.1 Main studies involving inflammatory markers and atrial fibrillation

Author/reference	Population and study design	Results
Aviles et al. (2003) [41]	Epidemiologic, cross-sectional study of 5,806 subjects, longitudinal study of 5,491	CRP associated with the presence of AF; CRP predicts patients at ↑ risk for future development of AF
Chung et al. (2001) [42]	Retrospective, observational case–control study, 131 patients with atrial arrhythmia and 71 controls	↑ CRP in AF, CRP ↑greater in persistent AF than paroxysmal AF
Dernellis and Panaretou (2004) [43]	Prospective case–control study, 50 patients with AF and 50 controls	↑ CRP in AF, CRP inversely related to successful cardioversion rate
Watanabe et al. (2005) [44]	Prospective, 50 AF patients	↑ CRP in PAF vs. control group; L-PAF had higher CRP levels than S-PAF; both S-PAF and L-PAF had larger LA diameter than control subjects; L-PAF > S-PAF in LA size
Asselbergs et al. (2005) [45]	Cross-sectional study, 8,501 patients	CRP and microalbuminuria are independent risk factors for AF; 2) both factors together represent a fourfold higher risk
Acevedo et al. (2003) [46]	Prospective, 109 patients with AF	↑ CRP in AF patients compared with control group at baseline; during follow-up, CRP in patients still in AF was significantly ↑ when compared with patients in SR
Psychari et al. (2005) [47]	Prospective, 90 patients with persistent and permanent AF and 46 controls	IL-6 and CRP participate in the evolution of AF; 2) LA size correlates with CRP and IL-6 levels
Conway et al. (2003) [39]	Cross-sectional observation study, 106 AF patients and 41 controls	↑ IL-6, CRP, and plasma viscosity, correlating to a prothrombotic state; ↑ IL-6 and CRP were independent predictors of stroke and composite end point of stroke or death

AF atrial fibrillation, *CRP* C-reactive protein, *IL* interleukin, *NSR* normal sinus rhythm, *PAF* paroxysmal atrial fibrillation, *LA* left appendage, *L-PAF* long paroxysmal atrial fibrillation, *SEC* spontaneous echo contrast, *S-PAF* short paroxysmal atrial fibrillation

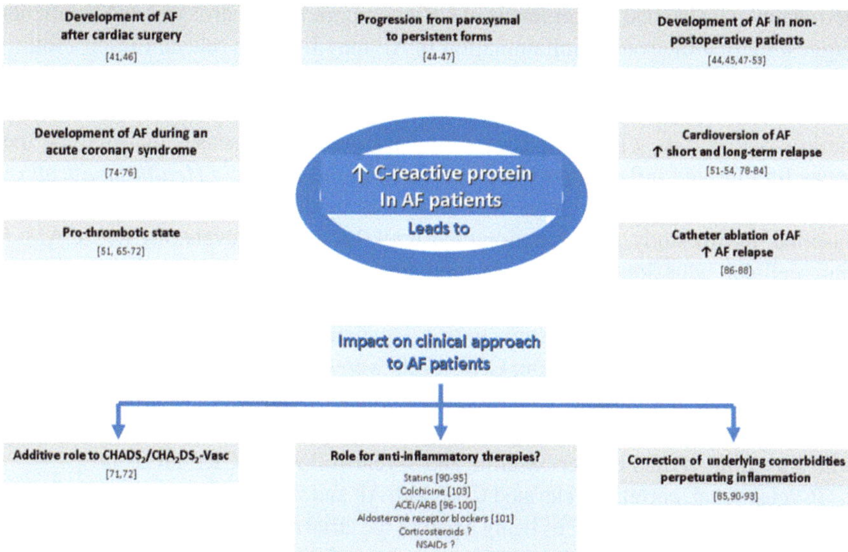

Fig. 2.3 Impact of elevated hsCRP levels in atrial fibrillation patients

CRP increase correlates with higher risk of cardiovascular events [49]. The exact mechanism beneath the association of CRP with AF is uncertain. This protein may be responsible for starting or perpetuating AF or can possibly just be a marker of underlying disease [42]. Figure 2.3 schematically summarizes the impact of elevated CRP levels in atrial fibrillation patients. It specifically binds to phosphatidylcholine on the membranes of myocardial cells activating the complement system and, in the presence of Ca^{2+} ions, leads to the formation of new molecular intermediaries responsible for cellular membrane dysfunction through changes in transmembrane ion transport [42]. CRP can also induce apoptotic loss of atrial myocytes due to calcium accumulation within atrial myocytes and may also play a role in the clearance of apoptotic atrial myocytes as an opsonin [42]. Since myocyte loss is typically accompanied by replacement fibrosis, inflammation provides substrate for AF development [42].

Serum CRP levels are significantly higher in patients with paroxysmal and chronic AF than in normal controls [50]. Similarly, CRP levels are higher in chronic AF patients than in paroxysmal AF patients [50]. The first investigation linking elevated CRP levels and AF was reported by Bruins and colleagues in the setting of cardiac surgery. They verified that patients who developed AF, mostly on the second/third postoperative day, concomitantly presented a peak elevation of CRP [51]. Years later in a small retrospective study, Aviles et al. demonstrated that patients who developed AF after major thoracic surgery had a nearly twofold increase in postoperative CRP levels in comparison with control subjects [41].

The relation between AF and CRP in non-postoperative patients was firstly reported by Chung and colleagues in a case–control study [42, 52]. CRP levels were more than twofold higher in patients with AF compared with controls. Patients with permanent AF also had higher levels of CRP compared with paroxysmal AF patients suggesting that the role of inflammation in AF may be more relevant in promoting persistence rather than initiating AF [42, 53].

Most of the previously reported studies consider patients with a moderate to high cardiovascular risk, with other coexisting cardiovascular diseases that may be the cause for elevated inflammatory markers [54]. In the *Women's Health Study*, all of the participating 24,734 women were free from cardiovascular disease and AF at baseline. In this study, inflammation measured through the levels of CRP, ICAM-1 (intercellular adhesion molecule 1), and fibrinogen was significantly associated with the risk of incident AF [54].

Acevedo et al. conducted a study with 130 patients with newly diagnosed nonvalvular AF [46]. In this population, CRP levels were predictors of AF at 30 days and at 1-year follow-up. Patients who reverted to sinus rhythm had lower baseline CRP levels. These low levels were kept during the first year of follow-up [46]. Patients who stayed in AF had higher baseline and 1-year follow-up CRP levels [46].

Psychari et al. correlated elevated CRP with AF and with left atrial size, suggesting a role for inflammation in AF as being a part of the atrial remodeling process and hence an important trigger [47]. Increased left atrial size and dysfunction were also correlated with higher CRP levels [44]. Watanabe et al. suggested that longer AF duration was associated with CRP elevation and an increased left atrial appendage diameter [44].

The association between AF and autoimmune diseases like Graves' and celiac disease and psoriasis suggests that AF could be a T-cell autoimmune disorder involving cytotoxic and helper T cells acting on His-Purkinje cells, which express contactin-2 [55]. Interestingly, this is one of the mechanisms known to be behind multiple sclerosis, and patients with this disease also have a higher incidence of atrial fibrillation [55]. However, since most of the His-Purkinje cells are in the ventricles, this relation is doubtful [55].

Interleukins and AF

The interleukin (IL) system is the main modulator of the inflammatory response [56]. IL-1β and IL-1Ra are the two major cytokines regulating inflammatory response. Genetic polymorphisms of IL-1 cluster genes are associated with increased risk of inflammatory and cardiovascular disease [56, 57]. VNTR (variable number tandem repeat) polymorphisms of the IL-1RN gene were associated with lone AF and also with several other chronic inflammatory diseases like ulcerative colitis, periodontitis, osteoarthritis, and gastric cancer [56, 57].

IL-6 is a cytokine involved in the synthesis of acute-phase proteins such as CRP. High plasma IL-6 levels have been correlated with the presence and duration of AF and increased left atrial diameter [58]. Both higher levels of IL-6 and several genetic polymorphisms, namely, in the promoter region of the IL-6 gene, were related with AF genesis in postoperative patients. Patients with AF and coronary disease had more frequently the CC genotype of 174G/C IL-6 polymorphisms. IL-8 (a cytokine that acts as a powerful chemoattractant for neutrophils) levels were also found to be elevated in AF patients [58].

Transforming Growth Factor

Transforming growth factor beta-1 (TGF-β1) is an important molecule promoting fibrosis in the liver, lung, kidney, pancreas, and other organs [59, 60]. It has been shown that it may also play an important role in the process of cardiac fibrosis, inflammation, and tissue remodeling organs [59, 60]. The TGF-β1 pathway is activated in AF; it can promote atrial fibrosis, inflammation, and tissue remodeling and then lead to tissue fibrosis [61].

Pentraxin 3

Pentraxin 3 is produced in local inflammatory lesions by various cells, namely, monocytes and macrophages, endothelial cells, vascular smooth muscle cells, fibroblasts, dendritic cells, and adipocytes [62]. Soeki et al. demonstrated that, in AF patients, the production of pentraxin 3 in the left atrium might reflect local inflammation; also in the GISSI-AF trial (*Use of Valsartan, an Angiotensin II AT1-Receptor Blocker in the Prevention of Atrial Fibrillation Recurrence*), higher concentrations of pentraxin 3 were detected in patients with AF, compared with those in sinus rhythm [62].

Oxidative Markers and Atrial Fibrillation

Emerging evidence implicates oxidative stress in the initiation and maintenance of AF. Oxidative stress promotes calcium overload and myocardial stunning alongside with decreased nitric oxide (NO) bioavailability [63]. Atrial redox balance results in a significant reduction in contractile response to β-adrenergic stimulation [63].

In experimental models, Carnes et al. have shown that AF induced in dogs decreases tissue ascorbate levels and increases protein nitration, a marker of oxidative stress [64]. These processes were accompanied by a decrease in the effective refractory period, changes consistent with atrial electrical remodeling [63]. Peroxynitrite and hydroxyl radicals, products of oxygen radical generation, have also been demonstrated in experimental models of AF. Experimental studies concluded that elevated levels of myeloperoxidase might favor the occurrence of AF in animals [64]. In experimental and clinical studies, a significant association between NADPH (nicotinamide adenine dinucleotide phosphate) oxidase-derived oxidative stress and AF was demonstrated [64].

Contrary to all these experimental data, in vivo studies have been difficult to perform because of the lack of reliable methods to quantify oxidative stress [65]. Oxidized glutathione and lipid peroxidation levels are elevated in coronary artery bypass surgery [65]. In patients after cardiac surgery, NADPH oxidase-derived ROS are overproduced in the right and left atria and are predictive of postoperative AF [63–65]. NADPH oxidase and dysfunctional nitric oxide synthase (NOS) contribute to superoxide production and may play an important role in atrial oxidative injury and electrophysiological remodeling in patients with AF [65].

Microalbuminuria, an abnormally increased urinary albumin excretion, is known to be an independent risk indicator for atherosclerotic disease. It is related with generalized vascular damage by lowering nitric oxide production. Asselbergs et al. demonstrated that elevated CRP and microalbuminuria were strongly associated with AF and that the combination of both markers led to a fourfold increase in the incidence of AF in the study population [45].

CRP and IL-6 in Atrial Fibrillation and Thrombosis

AF is associated with a prothrombotic or hypercoagulable state [66]. Thrombosis appears to be intimately related to inflammation. Some papers suggest that there is also an association between inflammatory status and thrombosis in patients with AF although the actual relation is not yet fully understood [66–68].

CRP and IL-6 can modify the procoagulant activity of inflammatory cells, promoting the synthesis of tissue factor, a major regulator of thrombosis [66–68]. IL-6 also increases platelet production and platelet sensitivity to thrombin, stimulates transcription of fibrinogen, and is linked to EC activation and damage. CRP has been found to be related to fibrinogen and plasma viscosity, and in the S-PAF III (*the Stroke Prevention in Atrial Fibrillation III*) study, patients with elevated CRP had a higher prevalence of stroke risk factors, vascular events, and total mortality [47].

Cianfrocca et al. conducted a cross-sectional study where 150 patients with AF underwent transesophageal echocardiography. Two groups were created according to the presence of dense spontaneous echo contrast in left atrium or appendage [67]. Patients with dense contrast had significantly more dilated left atria (diameter), lower left atrial appendage mean velocity, and higher levels of CRP. On multivariate analysis, left atrial appendage velocity and CRP were significantly associated with thrombus and/or dense contrast. Considering these data, the authors proposed that blood stasis and inflammation appear to constitute two major distinct components of thrombogenesis [67]. Thambidorai et al. investigated the relation between inflammation and thromboembolic risk factors in a population of 104 patients with AF [68]. Like other authors, they found that higher levels of CRP were related with anatomic and physiologic surrogates of thromboembolism such as thrombus, severe spontaneous echo contrast, and low left atrial appendage shear rate [47, 67–69]. Conversely, other authors reported that only IL-6 was an independent predictor of echocardiographic changes associated with stroke, although high plasma CRP showed a nonsignificant trend toward increased risk [70]. Maehama et al. studied the relation between inflammation and the presence or absence of left atrium thrombi in 190 patients with AF. CRP levels 1 week before the transesophageal echocardiography were independently associated with left atrial thrombi. A cutoff CRP value for identifying left atrial thrombus was 0.21 mg/dl (sensitivity, 84 %; specificity, 60 %; positive predictive value, 19 %; and negative predictive value, 97 %) [71].

A novel score (CATES), considering clinical risk factors, biomarkers (like CRP), and echocardiographic parameters proved to be better predictor of left atrial appendage thrombus than $CHADS_2$ and CHA_2DS_2-Vasc scores [72]. $CHADS_2$ is a commonly used score for embolic risk stratification. Patients in the high-risk group ($CHADS_2 > 3$) had significantly higher CRP levels than those in the intermediate ($CHADS_2 = 1$ and 2) and low risk ($CHADS_2 = 0$) (0.80 mg/dl, range 0.21–1.50, vs. 0.16 mg/dl, range 0.06–0.50, vs. 0.08 mg/dl, range 0.04–0.21, $p < 0.01$). The incidence of left atrial spontaneous echo contrast and left atrial thrombus increased alongside with increasing $CHADS_2$ score. During follow-up, the cardiovascular event-free survival was significantly lower in the high-risk group [70, 73]. According to these data, subsequent studies were performed using CRP associated with $CHADS_2$ score. This association allowed improved risk stratification beyond the $CHADS_2$ score, suggesting that CRP measurements might be included in the risk assessment of AF patients [73].

In a sub-study of the RE-LY (*Randomized Evaluation of Long-Term Anticoagulation Therapy*) trial, IL-6 was a predictor of stroke, and both IL-6 and CRP were associated with an increased risk of vascular death and cardiovascular events [74].

Atrial Fibrillation and Acute Coronary Syndrome

AF is a common complication of acute coronary syndromes (ACS), with an incidence of 10–20 % [75–77]. It is associated with increased intrahospital and long-term mortality since a rapid and irregular ventricular response may cause further impairment of coronary circulation [75]. According to Yoshizaki et al., AF in the early phase of ACS occurs a few days after the onset of the acute process, which is independently related to the activation of inflammatory pathways [76]. During this period, AF is usually sustained for only a short duration. In a sample of 259 patients with MI, AF was present in 14 % and occurred on day 2.4 ± 1.4 after admission. Patients with AF had significantly higher levels of CRP and white blood cell count [76]. Although it is widely known that CRP levels are increased during acute MI, CRP increase is more pronounced in patients with AF [76].

Inflammation in Atrial Fibrillation Cardioversion/Ablation

Cardioversion

Despite the use of antiarrhythmic agents for sinus rhythm maintenance, the majority of patients keep on presenting further episodes of AF [78]. AF relapse is common with studies indicating that 50–60 % of patients experience AF recurrence within the first month after cardioversion [78]. Relapse seems to be caused by electrical and/or structural remodeling of the atria and associated with older age, atrial dilation, and longer arrhythmia duration [78].

Several studies were conducted in order to assess the role of CRP as a predictor of short- and long-term risk of AF recurrence after electrical cardioversion. Although there is significant heterogeneity across studies, the majority suggests that higher levels of CRP associate with higher risk of AF relapse [44]. In a meta-analysis of seven prospective observational studies, increased baseline CRP levels were associated with greater risk of AF recurrence after successful cardioversion [79].

Lombardi and colleagues [80] studied 53 patients with preserved left ventricle ejection fraction and AF. Left atrial diameter and area and left atrial appendage emptying velocities were assessed pre-cardioversion. CRP levels were determined few hours before and 1 and 3 weeks after cardioversion. The authors concluded that none of the echocardiographic parameters reflecting atrial dysfunction predicted the outcome of the procedure. On the other hand, higher CRP levels (>3.0 mg/l) were significantly associated with AF recurrences [80].

Watanabe et al. reported that CRP levels were also predictors of successful cardioversion and found a significant positive correlation between CRP levels and the extent of coronary artery disease, smoking, diabetes, and AF duration [44]. In the same study, the authors observed an elevation in CRP levels after cardioversion only in patients with AF relapse, whereas CRP levels remained unchanged in subjects who were stable in sinus rhythm during the entire follow-up period [44]. Dernellis and Panaretou also demonstrated a strong relationship between CRP increase and the risk of AF recurrence. According to Fujiki et al., in long-standing persistent AF, lower levels of IL-6 and CRP appear to be associated with maintenance of sinus rhythm after pharmacological cardioversion [56].

Malouf et al. showed that CRP was independently associated with early AF recurrence in the first month after successful cardioversion [79]. Regarding only long-term recurrence, Loricchio's group followed a cohort of 102 consecutive patients with nonvalvular persistent AF who underwent electrical cardioversion and concluded that low CRP is associated with long-term maintenance of sinus rhythm [81]. Celebi et al. evaluated CRP levels both prior to and after cardioversion, predicting the long-term risk of AF relapse. CRP levels were significantly decreased in patients who remained in sinus rhythm at the end of the study and remained high throughout the follow-up in patients with an AF relapse [82].

Korantzopoulos et al., in a study of 60 patients, examined the time course of the inflammatory markers after cardioversion. Serial measurements of CRP, fibrinogen, and white blood cell count were performed on the first, third, and seventh day after cardioversion. Fibrinogen levels increased significantly in patients with AF relapse, and CRP values tended to decrease after cardioversion. This suggests that serial measurement of simple inflammatory indexes might be clinically useful in predicting success of cardioversion [83]. In a study by Ellinor et al., every 1 mg/dL increase in serum CRP was associated with a sevenfold increased risk of recurrent AF after cardioversion and a 12-fold increased risk of progression to permanent AF compared with controls [84].

All these findings are consistent with the concept that CRP levels may reflect structural changes associated with AF and that subclinical inflammation may be one of the most important factors in AF relapse. However, some papers present contradictory results. Deftereos et al. show no differences in CRP levels in peripheral venous blood samples of patients with and without AF recurrence, while IL-6 was higher in patients with recurrence [59]. In the population studied by Psychari et al., there was no association with several inflammatory markers like CRP and IL-6 and AF relapse [47]. Cosgrave et al. and Buob et al. measured CRP at baseline and few weeks after cardioversion and also found no differences in patients with AF recurrence [85].

Catheter Ablation

According to the most recent guidelines, catheter ablation is an effective alternative for the treatment of patients with symptomatic drug-refractory AF (class I recommendation, level A of evidence) [86]. Several studies were performed to examine the hypothesis of preexistent inflammatory response also increasing the likelihood of AF recurrence after catheter ablation (CA). Once again the results were inconsistent, but the majority favors the relation between inflammation and AF recurrence after catheter ablation [87].

In a study of 257 patients undergoing CA, only elevated CRP, left atrial diameter, and persistent AF duration were independent factors of relapse on multivariate analysis [87]. According to Liu et al., elevated CRP levels are associated with AF recurrence after CA of both paroxysmal and persistent AF patients [88].

The mechanisms of early and late AF recurrence after CA seem to differ. Early AF recurrence following ablation has been reported to be related to an acute inflammatory process secondary to massive tissue damage and profound inflammatory processes because of longer procedural time of aggressive radiofrequency ablation [89]. Regarding late AF recurrence, Lellouche et al. reported that a majority of patients (>90 %) with early recurrence will suffer also late recurrence, because of remodeling of atrial anatomy after catheter ablation [89].

The Use of Anti-inflammatory Drugs in Atrial Fibrillation

The importance of inflammation is supported also by studies assessing the use of statins in patients with AF. Statin therapy decreased the recurrence of AF after successful cardioversion [90]. Furthermore, statins also significantly reduced the risk of developing AF in patients with CAD regardless of the reduction in serum cholesterol [90]. This effect may be related with the pleiotropic effects of this family of drugs, which includes an anti-inflammatory action.

In a sub-analysis of the JUPITER trial, increasing levels of CRP were associated with an increased risk of incident AF, and the use of rosuvastatin significantly reduced that risk [91]. Out of the 17,120 patients without prior history of AF, each increasing tertile of baseline CRP was associated with a 36 % increase in the risk of developing AF, and the therapy with rosuvastatin was associated with a 27 % reduction in the relative risk of developing AF [91].

Table 2.2 Effects of statins in atrial fibrillation

Author/reference	Population and study design	Results
Kumagai et al. (2004) [93]	Blind, randomized, interventional canine, 10 control dogs and 10 dogs receiving atorvastatin	Atorvastatin-treated dogs had significantly ↓ CRP, ↓ duration of AF, and ↓ inflammation in atrial tissues
Siu et al. (2003) [94]	Retrospective, 62 patients with AF – 10 received statin and 52 in the control group	Patients treated with statin had ↓ recurrence of AF after EC than control subjects (40 % vs. 84 %)
Tveit et al. (2004) [92]	Prospective, randomized, longitudinal, open-label multicentre, interventional study, 114 patients randomized to pravastatin 40 mg versus none	Pravastatin therapy did not ↓ the recurrence rate of AF after electrical cardioversion
Young-Xu et al. (2003) [95]	Prospective, 449 patients with CAD	9 % of regular statin users developed AF, 10 % of intermittent statin users developed AF, and 15 % of non-statin users developed AF; statin effect was independent of lipid-lowering ability
Dernellis and Panaretou (2005) [43]	Prospective, 80 patients with AF randomized to 40 mg atorvastatin versus none	Treatment group had ↓ CRP levels at follow-up and ↓ number of PAF events; 65 % in treatment group had resolution of PAF

AF atrial fibrillation, *CRP* C-reactive protein, *EC* electrical cardioversion, *NSR* normal sinus rhythm, *PAF* paroxysmal atrial fibrillation

Dernellis et al. reported that CRP lowering with atorvastatin appears to be effective in suppressing paroxysms of AF during daily life in a significant proportion of patients [43]. However, Tveit et al. failed to demonstrate a reduction in the frequency of AF relapses after direct current cardioversion in patients treated with pravastatin 40 mg/day, compared with patients on standard therapy [92]. Table 2.2 presents the main studies using statins in AF.

Treatment with angiotensin-converting enzyme inhibitors (ACEI), angiotensin receptor blockers (ARB), aldosterone, and calcium channel blockers may also have a role in the prevention of AF onset and relapse [96–102]. All these drugs act by modifying inflammation. A recently published meta-analysis of 23 randomized controlled trials with 87,048 patients has shown that renin-angiotensin system inhibition reduces the incidence of AF by 33 % [96].

Large randomized studies investigated the effect of ACEI or ARB on the incidence of AF in patients with reduced left ventricular function. The conclusion from these trials is that the incidence of AF in patients treated with ACEI/ARB was significantly lower compared with the placebo group [97–100]. Table 2.3 presents the main studies using ACEI and ARB in AF.

Pretreatment with spironolactone in a ventricular tachypacing AF model reduced the amount of atrial fibrosis and inducibility of AF. Patients younger than 65 years with heart failure who received spironolactone were less likely to have atrial high-rate episodes compared with nonusers; however, the effect was not evident in older patients [101, 102].

Table 2.3 ACEI and ARB trials in atrial fibrillation

Authors/reference	Population and study design	Results
Pedersen et al. (1999) [97]	Retrospective analysis, 1,577 patients with reduced LVEF secondary to AMI	Trandolapril ↓ the incidence of AF
Vermes et al. (2003) [100]	Retrospective analysis, 391 patients with reduced LVEF or overt HF ACEI (enalapril) vs. placebo	ACEI significantly ↓ the risk of development of AF
Val-HeFT (2005) [98]	Prospective study with retrospective analysis 4,409 patients	Patients on ARB had ↓ incidence of AF
CHARM (2003) [99]	Prospective study with retrospective analysis 5,518 patients	ARB helps ↓ incidence of AF in both normal and depressed ejection fraction
SOLVD (2003) [100]	Prospective study with retrospective analysis 186 on enalapril and 188 in control	ACEI helps prevent AF in patients with depressed LV function

ACEI angiotensin-converting enzyme inhibitor, *Ang-II* angiotensin II, *AERP* atrial effective refractory period, *AF* atrial fibrillation, *ARB* angiotensin receptor blocker, *CHARM* candesartan in heart, *SOLVD* studies of left ventricular dysfunction, *Val-HeFT* Valsartan Heart Failure Trial

Colchicine after pulmonary vein isolation was used in a trial by Deftereos et al. After 3 months of treatment, the reported incidence of AF was significantly lower in patients receiving the drug. The authors proposed that the effect of colchicine was at least in part explained by its anti-inflammatory properties [103].

However, there is still controversy regarding the role of these agents in patients with AF. The European recommendations consider the use of ACEI/ARB for prevention of new-onset AF in patients with heart failure and reduced ejection fraction (class of recommendation IIA, level A of evidence) and in patients with arterial hypertension, particularly with left ventricular hypertrophy (class of recommendation IIA, level B of evidence). Statins should be considered for the prevention of new-onset AF after coronary artery bypass grafting, isolated or in combination with valvular interventions (class of recommendation IIA, level B of evidence) [86].

The recommendation and evidence are weaker, regarding the use of statins for the prevention of new-onset AF in patients with underlying heart disease, particularly heart failure (class of recommendation IIB, level B of evidence). Lastly, it is important to highlight that the use of ACEI, ARB, and statins, as upstream therapies, is not recommended for primary prevention of AF in patients without cardiovascular disease (class of recommendation III, level C of evidence) [86].

The 2014 American College of Cardiology/American Heart Association/Heart Rhythm Society guidelines on AF consider that an ACEI or ARB are reasonable for primary prevention of new-onset AF in patients with heart failure with reduced left ventricle function (class of recommendation IIA, level B of evidence) and may be considered for primary prevention of new-onset AF in the setting of arterial hypertension (class of recommendation IIB, level B of evidence). Regarding statin therapy, it may be reasonable for primary prevention of new-onset AF only after coronary artery surgery (class of recommendation IIB, level A of evidence) [104].

Therefore, quality and level of evidence and thus recommendations regarding modulation of inflammation through the use of several drug classes in patients with AF are mostly weak and result from small and non-randomized case–control studies. Further investigations, preferentially randomized controlled trials, should be carried out to confirm these preliminary results and provide further support to this approach.

Clinical Applications

The understanding of the pathogenesis of AF is still evolving, and inflammation has a significant impact on its pathogenesis. Whether inflammation is a cause or a consequence of the disease remains to be elucidated, but several mechanisms and biomarkers have been under investigation (Fig. 2.4), and clinical applications have been suggested. Table 2.4 illustrates the possible clinical applications of inflammatory biomarkers in patients with AF.

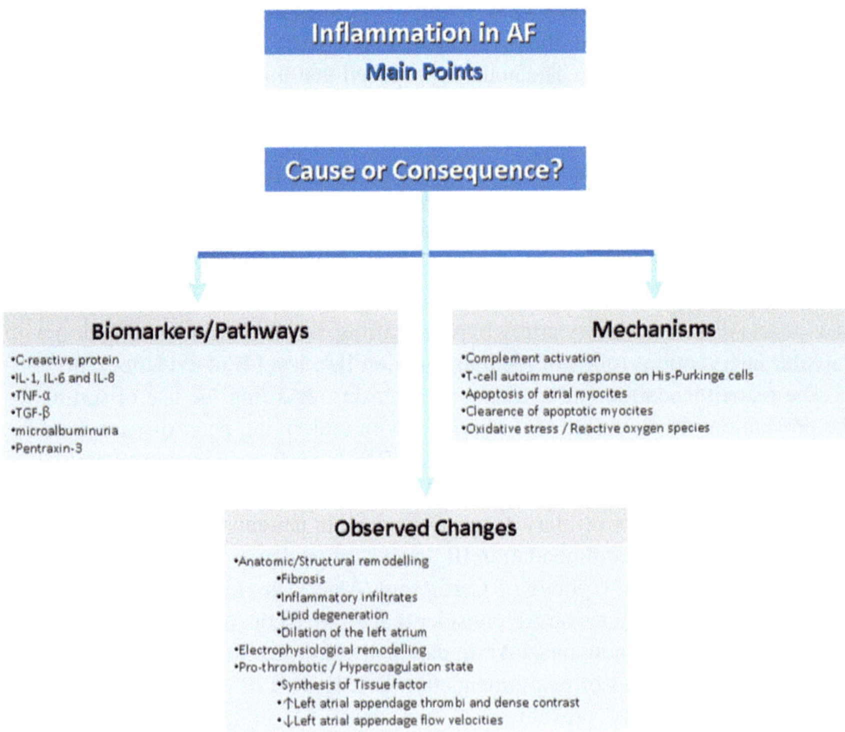

Fig. 2.4 Inflammation as cause or consequence of atrial fibrillation: biomarkers/pathways, mechanisms, and observed changes

Table 2.4 Prognostic role of inflammatory markers in atrial fibrillation

Inflammatory markers	Prognostic role in atrial fibrillation
CRP	Higher incidence of AF, incidence of LAF or paroxysmal AF, and recurrence after CV
	Higher risk of thromboembolic complications
IL-2	Predictor of early postoperative AF
	Low serum IL-2 levels on admission associated with successful CV
IL-6	Higher incidence of AF postoperation
	Higher incidence after catheter ablation
	Predictor of stroke and the composite end point of stroke and death in AF
Pentraxin 3	Higher levels in patients with AF
TGF-β	Promotes atrial fibrosis, inflammation, and tissue remodeling

AF atrial fibrillation, *CRP* C-reactive protein, *CV* cardioversion, *IL-2* interleukin 2, *IL-6* interleukin 6, *LAF* lone atrial fibrillation, *TGF-β* transforming growth factor beta

Take-Home Messages

- Atherosclerosis is now undoubtedly recognized as an inflammatory disease in which several immune cells (including monocytes–macrophages, T cells, NK cells, dendritic cells, and mast cells) participate.
- Inflammatory mediators, including acute-phase reactants, adhesion molecules, and cytokines, participate in atherosclerotic lesion initiation and progression as well as in plaque destabilization and rupture.
- A single inflammatory biomarker cannot alone reflect the inflammatory mechanisms underlying atherosclerosis development, but could help in improving diagnosis, prediction of risk and/or of mortality, and monitoring of therapeutic efficacy. At the moment, experimental and clinical data show that CRP is the best candidate to act as an inflammatory biomarker with clinical impact.
- Inflammation and oxidative stress play an important role in AF.
- Increased levels of CRP, IL-6, and other inflammatory markers have been found in patients with AF compared with controls in sinus rhythm.
- The rise of CRP levels may be responsible not only for the initiation but also for the perpetuation of AF.
- The success of cardioversion of AF is correlated with CRP and IL-6 levels.
- Anti-inflammatory agents may have a positive effect on the prevention and modulation of AF. However, the real effectiveness of these agents in this setting still remains to be conclusively proven.
- The coming years should prove fruitful in completing the picture of the role of inflammation in vascular and cardiac diseases, including atherosclerosis and AF, and in translating these concepts to clinical practice, thus improving human health.

Acknowledgments/Support The authors thank Portuguese Foundation for Science and Technology (FCT), COMPETE-FEDER and POPH/FSE, through the following support: PTDC/SAU-TOX/114253/2009 and UID/NEU/04539/2013 (CNC.IBILI).

References

1. Perk J, De Backer G, Gohlke H, Graham I, Reiner Z, Verschuren M, et al. European Guidelines on cardiovascular disease prevention in clinical practice (version 2012). The Fifth Joint Task Force of the European Society of Cardiology and Other Societies on Cardiovascular Disease Prevention in Clinical Practice (constituted by representatives of nine societies and by invited experts). Eur Heart J. 2012;33(13):1635–701.
2. Skalén K, Gustafsson M, Rydberg EK, Hulten LM, Wiklund O, Innerarity TL, et al. Subendothelial retention of atherogenic lipoproteins in early atherosclerosis. Nature. 2002;417:750–4.
3. Ait-Oufella H, Taleb S, Mallat Z, Tedgui A. Recent advances on the role of cytokines in atherosclerosis. Arterioscler Thromb Vasc Biol. 2011;31(5):969–79.
4. Lip GYH, Beevers DG. ABC of atrial fibrillation: history, epidemiology, and importance of atrial fibrillation. BMJ. 1995;311(7016):1361–93.
5. Lloyd-Jones DM, Want TJ, Leip EP, Larson MG, Levy D, Vasan RS, et al. Lifetime risk for development of atrial fibrillation: the Framingham Heart Study. Circulation. 2004;110(9):1042–6.
6. Pan M, Zhu JH, Jiang WP, Liu ZH, Li HM, Yu XH, et al. Inflammation: a possible pathogenic link to atrial fibrillation. Med Hypotheses. 2006;67(6):1305–7.
7. Wolf PA, Mitchell JB, Baker CS, Kannel WB, D'Agostino RB. Impact of atrial fibrillation on mortality, stroke, and medical costs. Arch Intern Med. 1998;158(3):229–34.
8. Wolf PA, Abbott RD, Kannel WB. Atrial fibrillation as an independent risk factor for stroke: the Framingham Study. Stroke. 1991;22:983–8.
9. Benjamin EJ, Levy D, Vaziri SM, D'Agostino RB, Belanger AJ, Wolf PA. Independent risk factors for atrial fibrillation in a population-based cohort: the Framingham Heart Study. JAMA. 1994;271(11):840–4.
10. Benjamin EJ, Wolf PA, D'Agostino RB, Silbershatz H, Kannel WB, Levy D. Impact of atrial fibrillation on the risk of death: the Framingham Heart Study. Circulation. 1998;98(10):946–52.
11. Patel AA, Ogden K, Veerman M, Mody SH, Nelson WW, Neil N. The economic burden to medicare of stroke events in atrial fibrillation populations with and without thromboprophylaxis. Popul Health Manag. 2014;17(3):159–65.
12. Lubitz SA, Benjamin EJ, Ellinor PT. Atrial fibrillation in congestive heart failure. Heart Fail Clin. 2010;6(2):187–200.
13. Savoia C, Schiffrin EL. Inflammation in hypertension. Curr Opin Nephrol Hypertens. 2006;15(2):152–8.
14. Paoletti R, Bolego C, Poli A, Cignarella A. Metabolic syndrome, inflammation and atherosclerosis. Vasc Health Risk Manag. 2006;2(2):145–52.
15. Hansson GK, Robertson AK, Söderberg-Nauclér C. Inflammation and atherosclerosis. Annu Rev Pathol. 2006;1:297–329.
16. Aukrust P, Halvorsen B, Yndestad A, Ueland T, Øie E, Otterdal K, et al. Chemokines and cardiovascular risk. Arterioscler Thromb Vasc Biol. 2008;28(11):1909–19.
17. Weber C, Fraemohs L, Dejana E. The role of junctional adhesion molecules in vascular inflammation. Nat Rev Immunol. 2007;7(6):467–77.

18. Amorino GP, Hoover RL. Interactions of monocytic cells with human endothelial cells stimulate monocytic metalloproteinase production. Am J Pathol. 1998;152(1):199–207.
19. Hansson GK, Libby P, Schönbeck U, Yan ZQ. Innate and adaptive immunity in the pathogenesis of atherosclerosis. Circ Res. 2002;91(4):281–91.
20. Packard RR, Libby P. Inflammation in atherosclerosis: from vascular biology to biomarker discovery and risk prediction. Clin Chem. 2008;54(1):24–38.
21. Han CI, Campbell GR, Campbell JH. Circulating bone marrow cells can contribute to neointimal formation. J Vasc Res. 2001;38:113–9.
22. Hansson GK. Inflammatory mechanisms in atherosclerosis. J Thromb Haemost. 2009;7 Suppl 1:328–31.
23. Libby P. Inflammation in atherosclerosis. Arterioscler Thromb Vasc Biol. 2012;32(9):2045–51.
24. Badimon L, Storey RF, Vilahur G. Update on lipids, inflammation and atherothrombosis. Thromb Haemost. 2011;105 Suppl 1:S34–42.
25. Mach F, Schonbeck U, Sukhova GK, Bourcier T, Bonnefoy JY, Pober JS, et al. Functional CD40 ligand is expressed on human vascular endothelial cells, smooth muscle cells, and macrophages: implications for CD40-CD40 ligand signaling in atherosclerosis. Proc Natl Acad Sci U S A. 1997;94(5):1931–6.
26. Libby P, Okamoto Y, Rocha VZ, Folco E. Inflammation in atherosclerosis: transition from theory to practice. Circ J. 2010;74(2):213–20.
27. Yousuf O, Mohanty BD, Martin SS, Joshi PH, Blaha MJ, Nasir K, et al. High-sensitivity C-reactive protein and cardiovascular disease: a resolute belief or an elusive link? J Am Coll Cardiol. 2013;62(5):397–408.
28. Ridker PM, Cushman M, Stampfer MJ, Tracy RP, Hennekens CH. Inflammation, aspirin, and the risk of cardiovascular disease in apparently healthy men. N Engl J Med. 1997;336(14):973–9.
29. Pearson TA, Mensah GA, Alexander RW, Anderson JL, Cannon 3rd RO, Criqui M, et al. Markers of inflammation and cardiovascular disease: application to clinical and public health practice: a statement for healthcare professionals from the Centers for Disease Control and Prevention and the American Heart Association. Circulation. 2003;107(3):499–511.
30. Ridker PM, Buring JE, Rifai N, Cook NR. Development and validation of improved algorithms for the assessment of global cardiovascular risk in women: the Reynolds risk score. JAMA. 2007;297(6):611–9.
31. Ridker PM, Danielson E, Fonseca FA, Genest J, Gotto Jr AM, Kastelein JJ, et al. Rosuvastatin to prevent vascular events in men and women with elevated C-reactive protein. N Engl J Med. 2008;359(21):2195–207.
32. Ridker PM, Danielson E, Fonseca FA, Genest J, Gotto Jr AM, Kastelein JJ, et al. Reduction in C-reactive protein and LDL cholesterol and cardiovascular event rates after initiation of rosuvastatin: a prospective study of the JUPITER trial. Lancet. 2009;373(9670):1175–82.
33. Malouf JF, Kanagala R, Al Atawi FO, Rosales AG, Davison DE, Murali NS, et al. High sensitivity C-reactive protein: a novel predictor for recurrence of atrial fibrillation after successful cardioversion. J Am Coll Cardiol. 2005;46(7):1284–7.
34. Wijffels M, Kirchhof C, Dorland R, Allessie MA. Atrial fibrillation begets atrial fibrillation. A study in awake chronically instrumented goats. Circulation. 1995;92(7):1954–68.
35. Garrey WE. The nature of fibrillary contraction of the heart: its relation to tissue mass and form. Am J Physiol. 1964;33:397–414.
36. Haïssaguerre M, Jaïs P, Shah DC, Takahashi A, Hocini M, Quiniou G, et al. Spontaneous initiation of atrial fibrillation by ectopic beats originating in the pulmonary veins. N Engl J Med. 1998;339(10):659–66.
37. Nakamura Y, Nakamura K, Fukushima-Kusano K, Ohta K, Matsubara H, Hamuro T, et al. Tissue factor expression in atrial endothelia associated with nonvalvular atrial fibrillation: possible involvement in intracardiac thrombogenesis. Thromb Res. 2003;111(3):137–42.

38. Frustaci A, Chimenti C, Bellocci F, Morgante E, Russo MA, Maseri A. Histological substrate of atrial biopsies in patients with lone atrial fibrillation. Circulation. 1997;96(4):1180–4.
39. Conway DS, Buggins P, Hughes E, Lip GY. Prognostic significance of raised plasma levels of interleukin-6 and C-reactive protein in atrial fibrillation. Am Heart J. 2004;148(3):462–6.
40. Toutouzas K, Synetos A, Drakopoulou M, Stefanadi E, Tousoulis D, Lerakis S, et al. The role of inflammation in atrial fibrillation: a myth or a fact? Am J Med Sci. 2009;338(6):494–9.
41. Aviles RJ, Martin DO, Apperson-Hansen C, Houghtaling PL, Rautaharju P, Kronmal RA, et al. Inflammation as a risk factor for atrial fibrillation. Circulation. 2003;108(24):3006–10.
42. Chung M, Martin D, Sprecher D, Wazni O, Kanderian A, Carnes CA, et al. C-reactive protein elevation in patients with atrial arrhythmias: inflammatory mechanisms and persistence of atrial fibrillation. Circulation. 2001;104(24):2886–91.
43. Dernellis J, Panaretou M. Effect of C-reactive protein reduction on paroxysmal atrial fibrillation. Am Heart J. 2005;150(5):1064.
44. Watanabe T, Takeishi Y, Hirono O, Itoh M, Matsui M, Nakamura K, et al. C-reactive protein elevation predicts the occurrence of atrial structural remodeling in patients with paroxysmal atrial fibrillation. Heart Vessels. 2005;20(2):45–9.
45. Asselbergs FW, van den Berg MP, Diercks GF, van Gilst WH, van Veldhuisen DJ. C-reactive protein and microalbuminuria are associated with atrial fibrillation. Int J Cardiol. 2005;98(1):73–7.
46. Acevedo M, Corbalán R, Braun S, Pereira J, Navarrete C, Gonzalez I. C-reactive protein and atrial fibrillation: "evidence for the presence of inflammation in the perpetuation of the arrhythmia". Int J Cardiol. 2006;108(3):326–31.
47. Psychari SN, Apostolou TS, Sinos L, Hamodraka E, Liakos G, Kremastinos DT. Relation of elevated C-reactive protein and interleukin-6 levels to left atrial size and duration of episodes in patients with atrial fibrillation. Am J Cardiol. 2005;95(6):764–7.
48. Aguiar FJ, Ferreira-Júnior M, Sales MM, Cruz-Neto LM, Fonseca LA, Sumita NM, et al. C-reactive protein: clinical applications and proposals for a rational use. Rev Assoc Med Bras. 2013;59(1):85–92.
49. Hernández Madrid A. Proteína C reactiva y fibrilación auricular. Un viejo marcador en busca de un nuevo sitio. Rev Esp Cardiol. 2006;59:94–8.
50. Li SB, Yang F, Jing L, Ma J, Jia YD, Dong SY, et al. Myeloperoxidase and risk of recurrence of atrial fibrillation after catheter ablation. J Investig Med. 2013;61(4):722–7.
51. Bruins P, te Velthuis H, Yazdanbakhsh AP, Jansen PG, van Hardevelt FW, de Beaumont EM, et al. Activation of the complement system during and after cardiopulmonary bypass surgery: postsurgery activation involves C-reactive protein and is associated with postoperative arrhythmia. Circulation. 1997;96(10):3542–8.
52. Dernellis J, Panaretou M. Relationship between C-reactive protein concentrations during glucocorticoid therapy and recurrent atrial fibrillation. Eur Heart J. 2004;25(13):1100–7.
53. Engelmann MDM, Svendsen JH. Inflammation in the genesis and perpetuation of atrial fibrillation. Eur Heart J. 2005;26(20):2083–92.
54. Conen D, Ridker PM, Everett BM, Tedrow UB, Rose L, Cook NR, et al. A multimarker approach to assess the influence of inflammation on the incidence of atrial fibrillation in women. Eur Heart J. 2010;31(14):1730–6.
55. Schairer DO, Levis WR. Atrial fibrillation: an inflammatory and autoimmune disorder. Heart Rhythm. 2012;9(2):e2.
56. Fujiki A, Sakamoto T, Nishida K, Mizumaki K, Inoue H. Relation of interleukin-6 and C-reactive protein levels to sinus maintenance after pharmacological cardioversion in persistent atrial fibrillation. J Cardiovasc Pharmacol. 2007;50(3):264–6.
57. Gungor B, Ekmekci A, Arman A, et al. Assessment of interleukin-1 gene cluster polymorphisms in lone atrial fibrillation: new insight into the role of inflammation in atrial fibrillation. Pacing Clin Electrophysiol. 2013;36(10):1220–7.

58. Patel P, Dokainish H, Tsai P, Lakkis N. Update on the association of inflammation and atrial fibrillation. J Cardiovasc Electrophysiol. 2010;21(9):1064–70.
59. Deftereos S, Giannopoulos G, Kossyvakis C, Raisakis K, Angelidis C, Efremidis M, et al. Association of post-cardioversion transcardiac concentration gradient of soluble tumor necrosis factor-related apoptosis-inducing ligand (sTRAIL) and inflammatory biomarkers to atrial fibrillation recurrence. Clin Biochem. 2013;46(12):1020–5.
60. Hermida J, Lopez FL, Montes R, Matsushita K, Astor BC, Alonso A. Usefulness of high-sensitivity C-reactive protein to predict mortality in patients with atrial fibrillation (from the atherosclerosis risk in communities [ARIC] study). Am J Cardiol. 2012;109(1):95–9.
61. Mira YE, Muhuyati, Lu WH, He PY, Liu ZQ, Yang YC. TGF-β1 signal pathway in the regulation of inflammation in patients with atrial fibrillation. Asian Pac J Trop Med. 2013;6(12):999–1003.
62. Soeki T, Bando S, Uematsu E, Matsuura T, Niki T, Ise T, et al. Pentraxin 3 is a local inflammatory marker in atrial fibrillation. Heart Vessels. 2014;29(5):653–8.
63. Li J, Solus J, Chen Q, Rho YH, Milne G, Stein CM, et al. The role of inflammation and oxidative stress in atrial fibrillation. Heart Rhythm. 2010;7(4):438–44.
64. Kim Y, Guzik T, Zhang Y, Zhang MH, Kattach H, Ratnatunga C, et al. A myocardial Nox2 containing NAD(P)H oxidase contributes to oxidative stress in human atrial fibrillation. Circ Res. 2005;97(7):629–36.
65. Lip GY, Patel JV, Hughes E, Hart RG. High-sensitivity C-reactive protein and soluble CD40 ligand as indices of inflammation and platelet activation in 880 patients with nonvalvular atrial fibrillation: relationship to stroke risk factors, stroke risk stratification schema, and prognosis. Stroke. 2007;38(4):1229–37.
66. Lip GY. Does atrial fibrillation confer a hypercoagulable state? Lancet. 1995;346(8986):1313–4.
67. Cianfrocca C, Loricchio ML, Pelliccia F, Pasceri V, Auriti A, Bianconi L, et al. C-reactive protein and left atrial appendage velocity are independent determinants of the risk of thrombogenesis in patients with atrial fibrillation. Int J Cardiol. 2010;142(1):22–8.
68. Thambidorai SK, Parakh K, Martin DO, Shah TK, Wazni O, Jasper SE, et al. Relation of C-reactive protein correlates with risk of thromboembolism in patients with atrial fibrillation. Am J Cardiol. 2004;94(6):805–7.
69. Thambidorai SK, Murray RD, Parakh K, Shah TK, Black IW, Jasper SE, et al. Utility of transesophageal echocardiography in identification of thrombogenic milieu in patients with atrial fibrillation (an ACUTE ancillary study). Am J Cardiol. 2005;96(78):935–41.
70. Gage BF, Waterman AD, Shannon W, et al. Validation of clinical classification schemes for predicting stroke: results from the National Registry of Atrial Fibrillation. JAMA. 2001;285:2864–70.
71. Maehama T, Okura H, Imai K, Saito K, Yamada R, Koyama T, et al. Systemic inflammation and left atrial thrombus in patients with non-rheumatic atrial fibrillation. J Cardiol. 2010;56(1):118–24.
72. Providência R, Faustino A, Paiva L, Trigo J, Botelho A, Nascimento J, et al. Cardioversion safety in patients with nonvalvular atrial fibrillation: which patients can be spared transesophageal echocardiography? Blood Coagul Fibrinolysis. 2012;23(7):597–602.
73. Maehama T, Okura H, Imai K, Yamada R, Obase K, Saito K, et al. Usefulness of CHADS2 score to predict C-reactive protein, left atrial blood stasis, and prognosis in patients with nonrheumatic atrial fibrillation. Am J Cardiol. 2010;106(4):535–8.
74. Aulin JK, Ezekowitz MD, Andersson U, Connolly SJ, Huber K, Reilly PA, et al. Interleukin-6 and C-reactive protein and risk for death and cardiovascular events in patients with atrial fibrillation. J Am Coll Cardiol. 2011;57(14s1):E91.
75. Crenshaw BS, Ward SR, Granger CB, Stebbins AL, Topol EJ, Califf RM. Atrial fibrillation in the setting of acute myocardial infarction: the GUSTO-I experience. Global utilization of streptokinase and TPA for occluded coronary arteries. J Am Coll Cardiol. 1997;30(2):406–13.

76. Yoshizaki T, Umetani K, Ino Y, Takahashi S, Nakamura M, Seto T, et al. Activated inflammation is related to the incidence of atrial fibrillation in patients with acute myocardial infarction. Intern Med. 2012;51(12):1467–71.
77. The Emerging Risk Factors Collaboration, Kaptoge S, Di Angelantonio E, Lowe G, Pepys MB, Thompson SG, et al. C-reactive protein concentration and risk of coronary heart disease, stroke and mortality: an individual participant meta-analysis. Lancet. 2010;375(9709):132–40.
78. Liu T, Li G, Li L, Korantzopoulos P. Association between C-reactive protein and recurrence of atrial fibrillation after successful electrical cardioversion: a meta-analysis. J Am Coll Cardiol. 2007;49(15):1642–8.
79. Wu N, Xu B, Xiang Y, Wu L, Zhang Y, Ma X, et al. Association of inflammatory factors with occurrence and recurrence of atrial fibrillation: a meta-analysis. Int J Cardiol. 2013;169(1):62–72.
80. Lombardi F, Tundo F, Belletti S, Mantero A, Melzi D'eril GV. C-reactive protein but not atrial dysfunction predicts recurrences of atrial fibrillation after cardioversion in patients with preserved left ventricular function. J Cardiovasc Med (Hagerstown). 2008;9(6):581–8.
81. Loricchio ML, Cianfrocca C, Pasceri V, Bianconi L, Auriti A, Calo L, et al. Relation of C-reactive protein to long-term risk of recurrence of atrial fibrillation after electrical cardioversion. Am J Cardiol. 2007;99(10):1421–4.
82. Celebi OO, Celebi S, Canbay A, Ergun G, Aydogdu S, Diker E. The effect of sinus rhythm restoration on high-sensitivity C-reactive protein levels and their association with long-term atrial fibrillation recurrence after electrical cardioversion. Cardiology. 2011;118(3):168–74.
83. Korantzopoulos P, Kolettis TM, Kountouris E, Siogas K, Goudevenos JA. Variation of inflammatory indexes after electrical cardioversion of persistent atrial fibrillation. Is there an association with early recurrence rates? Int J Clin Pract. 2005;59(8):881–5.
84. Ellinor PT, Low A, Patton KK, Shea MA, MacRae CA. C-reactive protein in lone atrial fibrillation. Am J Cardiol. 2006;97(9):1346–50.
85. Cosgrave J, Foley JB, Bahadur K, Bennett K, Crean P, Walsh MJ. Inflammatory markers are not associated with outcomes following elective external cardioversion. Int J Cardiol. 2006;110(3):373–7.
86. Camm AJ, Lip GY, De Caterina R, Savelieva I, Atar D, Hohnloser SH, et al. 2012 focused update of the ESC Guidelines for the management of atrial fibrillation: an update of the 2010 ESC Guidelines for the management of atrial fibrillation developed with the special contribution of the European Heart Rhythm Association. Eur Heart J. 2012;33(21):2719–47.
87. Kurotobi T, Iwakura K, Inoue K, Kimura R, Okamura A, Koyama Y, et al. A pre-existent elevated C-reactive protein is associated with the recurrence of atrial tachyarrhythmias after catheter ablation in patients with atrial fibrillation. Europace. 2010;12:1213–8.
88. Liu J, Fang PH, Dibs S, Hou Y, Li XF, Zhang S. High-sensitivity C-reactive protein as a predictor of atrial fibrillation recurrence after primary circumferential pulmonary vein isolation. Pacing Clin Electrophysiol. 2011;34(4):398–406.
89. Jiang Z, Dai L, Song Z, Li H, Shu M. Association between C-reactive protein and atrial fibrillation recurrence after catheter ablation: a meta-analysis. Clin Cardiol. 2013;36(9):548–54.
90. Issac TT, Dokainish H, Lakkis NM. Role of inflammation in initiation and perpetuation of atrial fibrillation: a systematic review of the published data. J Am Coll Cardiol. 2007;20(21):2021–8.
91. Peña JM, MacFadyen J, Glynn RJ, Ridker PM. High-sensitivity C-reactive protein, statin therapy, and risks of atrial fibrillation: an exploratory analysis of the JUPITER trial. Eur Heart J. 2012;33(4):531–7.
92. Tveit A, Grundtvig M, Gundersen T, Vanberg P, Semb AG, Holt E, et al. Analysis of pravastatin to prevent recurrence of atrial fibrillation after electrical cardioversion. Am J Cardiol. 2004;93(6):780–2.
93. Kumagai K, Nakashima H, Saku K. The HMG-CoA reductase inhibitor atorvastatin prevents atrial fibrillation by inhibiting inflammation in a canine sterile pericarditis model. Cardiovasc Res. 2004;62(1):105–11.

94. Siu CW, Lau CP, Tse HF. Prevention of atrial fibrillation recurrence by statin therapy in patients with lone atrial fibrillation after successful cardioversion. Am J Cardiol. 2003;92(11):1343–5.
95. Young-Xu Y, Jabbour S, Goldberg R, Blatt CM, Graboys T, Bilchik B, Ravid S. Usefulness of statin drugs in protecting against atrial fibrillation in patients with coronary artery disease. Am J Cardiol. 2003;92(12):1379–83.
96. Healey JS, Baranchuk A, Crystal E, Morillo CA, Garfinkle M, Yusuf S, et al. Prevention of atrial fibrillation with angiotensin-converting enzyme inhibitors and angiotensin receptor blockers: a meta-analysis. J Am Coll Cardiol. 2005;45(11):1832–9.
97. Pedersen O, Bagger H, Kober L, Torp-Pedersen C. Trandolapril reduces the incidence of atrial fibrillation after acute myocardial infarction in patients with left ventricular dysfunction. Circulation. 1999;100(4):376–80.
98. Maggioni AP, Latini R, Carson PE, Singh SN, Barlera S, Glazer R, et al. Valsartan reduces the incidence of atrial fibrillation in patients with heart failure: results from the Valsartan Heart Failure Trial (Val-HeFT). Am Heart J. 2005;149(3):548–57.
99. Pfeffer MA, Swedberg K, Granger CB, Held P, McMurray JJ, Michelson EL, et al. Effects of candesartan on mortality and morbidity in patients with chronic heart failure: the CHARM-Overall programme. Lancet. 2003;362(9386):759–66.
100. Vermes E, Tardif JC, Bourassa MG, Racine N, Levesque S, White M, et al. Enalapril decreases the incidence of atrial fibrillation in patients with left ventricular dysfunction: insight from the Studies Of Left Ventricular Dysfunction (SOLVD) trials. Circulation. 2003;107(23):2926–31.
101. Yang SS, Han W, Zhou HY, Dong G, Wang BC, Huo H, et al. Effects of spironolactone on electrical and structural remodeling of atrium in congestive heart failure dogs. Chin Med J (Engl). 2008;121(1):38–42.
102. Brinkley DM, Chen J. Effect of spironolactone on atrial fibrillation in patients with heart failure. Heart Rhythm. 2010;7:S262.
103. Marcus GM, Hsu JC. Colchicine after pulmonary vein isolation to prevent the early recurrence of atrial fibrillation, mollifying an inflammatory response? J Am Coll Cardiol. 2012;60(18):1797–8.
104. January CT, Wann LS, Alpert JS, Calkins H, Cleveland Jr JC, Cigarroa JE, et al. Practice Guidelines and the Heart Rhythm Society Report of the American College of Cardiology/American Heart Association Task Force on 2014 AHA/ACC/HRS Guideline for the management of patients with atrial fibrillation. Circulation. 2014;2014(3):735–1097.

Chapter 3
Diabetes Mellitus and Metabolic Syndrome

Eduardo Ortega, Leticia Martín-Cordero, Pablo M. Garcia-Roves, Adam J. Chicco, Alba Gonzalez-Franquesa, and Daniela Marado

Abstract Type 2 diabetes mellitus and metabolic syndrome are two highly prevalent clinical entities in our population and threaten to become a true pandemic. While there are still gaps in medical knowledge about the pathophysiological mechanisms leading to the development of both conditions, a significant effort has been made to study them in detail. Inflammation has been recognized as a major player in all this, and the advancement of knowledge in this area has been fruitful. This chapter will address the inflammatory mechanisms underlying these entities, starting with a more mechanistic and molecular perspective and ending in a more clinical setting.

Keywords Type 2 diabetes mellitus • Metabolic syndrome • Inflammation • Mediators of inflammation • Insulin resistance • Cardiometabolic risk

The coexistence of a disturbed glucose and insulin metabolism, mild dyslipidemia, overweight and abdominal fat distribution, and arterial hypertension in an individual

E. Ortega, Ph.D. (✉)
Department of Physiology (Immunophysiology Research Group), Faculty of Sciences, University of Extremadura, Avda Elvas, s/n, 06071 Badajoz, Spain
e-mail: orincon@unex.es

L. Martín-Cordero, Ph.D.
Department of Nursing (Immunophysiology Research Group), University of Extremadura, Badajoz, Spain

P.M. Garcia-Roves, Ph.D.
Department of Physiological Sciences II, Faculty of Medicine, University of Barcelona, L'Hospitalet Llobregat, Spain

A.J. Chicco, Ph.D.
Department of Health and Exercise and Biomedical Sciences, Colorado State University, Fort Collins, CO, USA

A. Gonzalez-Franquesa, M.Sc., Ph.D.
Diabetes and Obesity Laboratory, Institut d'Investigacions Biomèdiques August Pi I Sunyer (IDIBAPS), Barcelona, Spain

D. Marado, M.D.
Department of Internal Medicine – B, Centro Hospitalar e Universitário de Coimbra, Coimbra, Portugal

© Springer International Publishing Switzerland 2015

F. Palavra et al. (eds.), *Biomarkers of Cardiometabolic Risk, Inflammation and Disease*, DOI 10.1007/978-3-319-16018-4_3

subject may be associated with subsequent development of type 2 diabetes (T2D) and cardiovascular events. This has given rise to the concept of metabolic syndrome (MetS), insulin resistance being considered the underlying abnormality of this constellation of problems. Both T2D and MetS are extremely prevalent clinical entities in our society, and the fact is that they can become, in the short term, a true pandemic. The pathogenesis of these conditions is not yet fully understood, but medical knowledge has been advancing significantly in this area, in recent years, and more and more mediators and mechanisms are called into the field as players in these complex processes. Inflammation has been implicated as an important player in the pathogenesis of these conditions, and knowledge that has been generated only reinforces its ubiquitous and crucial character, making it an extremely interesting target for future therapeutic developments. This chapter will focus on the inflammatory mechanisms underlying T2D and MetS, starting with a more mechanistic perspective and ending with a clinical view, highlighting all biomarkers that, at least theoretically, can be useful in the assessment of cardiometabolic risk for these patients.

Inflammation and Stress in Diabetes Mellitus and Metabolic Syndrome

Metabolic syndrome (MetS), or insulin resistance syndrome, is a metabolic disorder associated with obesity that involves risk factors for T2D and arteriosclerosis, with the concomitant increased risk of cardiovascular events [1]. A close link between metabolism, stress, and immunity explains the association of MetS with a state of "chronic low-grade inflammation" [2, 3], a condition that has been defined by a two- to threefold increase in the systemic concentration of tumor necrosis factor alpha (TNF-α), interleukin (IL)-1 beta (IL-1β), IL-6, IL-1 receptor antagonist (IL-1ra), soluble TNF receptors (sTNF-R), and C-reactive protein (CRP) [4]. These molecules are known to play a role in the pathobiology of MetS-associated disorders, such as obesity, insulin resistance (IR), coronary heart disease, T2D, and arterial hypertension [2]. Thus, obesity and T2D are associated with an altered interaction between the metabolic and the immune systems, which has recently been termed "immunometabolism" [5–8]. In fact, much evidence suggests that a crosstalk interaction between inflammatory-signaling and insulin-signaling pathways causes both metabolic IR and endothelial dysfunction and that in MetS these synergize to predispose to cardiovascular disorders (CVD) [6].

Inflammatory and Stress-Induced Neuroendocrine Mediators Are Altered in Metabolic Syndrome

Low-Grade Systemic Inflammation and Metabolic Syndrome

Many studies have shown that abdominal obesity is associated with systemic low-grade inflammation leading to IR and MetS. Thus, systemic inflammatory biomarkers could predict development of T2D and CVD in the general population [7].

Studies on humans have shown that adipose tissue produces and releases a great number of bioactive proteins, collectively known as adipokines [8], some of which are increased in obese or overweight individuals. The first molecular link recognized between inflammation and obesity was TNF-α, since this inflammatory cytokine is overexpressed in the adipose tissues of obese rodent models, and it is also overproduced in the adipose and muscle tissues of obese humans [9]. Obese humans also have increased circulating levels of TNF-α, together with elevated concentrations of IL-6, IL-8, IL-10, IL-18, and CRP (reviewed in [10]). However, Bastard et al. suggested that adipose tissue is not directly implicated in the increased circulating TNF-α levels in obese humans, hypothesizing that other mechanisms involving, for example, a systemic effect of leptin may induce TNF-α secretion by other cell types [9, 11]. In fact, given the relationship that leptin has with acute and chronic inflammation, this adipokine has been proposed as a valuable biomarker for predicting acute inflammation in individuals with both obesity and diabetes [12].

The multifunctional cytokine IL-6 is clearly involved in the regulation of metabolism, stress, and the immune system but is still the subject of major physiological controversies. It has been suggested that circulating IL-6 plays an important role in the development of IR and atherosclerosis through its effects on metabolism – reducing hepatic insulin sensitivity and glucose uptake by adipocytes and causing raised plasma insulin levels, hyperglycemia, and hyperlipidemia (reviewed by Eder et al. [13]). However, other studies find arguments for IL-6 having a lipolytic role, with its participation in lipolysis and fat oxidation [14]. The controversy was sharpened with the observation that IL-6 knockout mice develop mature-onset obesity, with hypertriglyceridemia, glucose intolerance, and other features of MetS, while a subsequent study observed no such phenomenon, probably because the comparison was made with different control strains [13].

IL-6 can also contribute indirectly (but no less importantly) to the T2D and CVD risk associated with MetS via the inhibition of the release of TNF-α by immune cells and also by stimulating the release of CRP from hepatic and adipose tissues. Elevated levels of CRP (the main circulating inflammatory molecule) are also particularly clearly related with MetS and with increased risk for CVD. Although most current definitions do not include inflammation as a criterion in defining MetS, it has been strongly suggested that the associations between CRP and the factors defining MetS are not causal [15]. Therefore, it is still necessary to examine the relationships between reductions in inflammatory biomarkers such as CRP, improved insulin sensitivity, and primary endpoints including the outcomes of CVD and the incidence of diabetes [6]. Pischon et al. [16] confirmed that people with MetS show higher levels of CRP than healthy people, and there can also be a link not only with obesity, IR, and diabetes but also with hypertension and low high-density lipoprotein cholesterol (HDL-C) levels. Studies in vitro have shown that aggregated CRP binds to low-density lipoprotein (LDL) and very low-density lipoprotein (VLDL), leading to the activation of complement and to the initiation of coagulation, thus explaining in part the connection between CVD and CRP [17]. In fact, it is well known that mechanisms reducing inflammation improve endothelial dysfunction and decrease IR in atherosclerosis, coronary heart disease, and hypertension in the context of insulin-resistant states (including diabetes, obesity, and MetS) [6].

Dysregulation Between the Inflammatory and Stress Response in the Metabolic Syndrome

It is currently accepted that neuroendocrine-immune disorders can play a role in obesity, arterial hypertension, and IR and that neuroendocrine-immune dysfunction is associated either with abnormalities in the inflammatory response or with the local overactivity of pro-inflammatory factors [18]. Neuroadrenergic dysfunction, including increased resting activity in the sympathetic nervous system (SNS), is a recognized feature of obesity in MetS, contributing to its pathophysiology and clinical prognosis [19]. It is well known that noradrenaline (NA) is involved in metabolic regulation, and it is also true that almost all the mechanisms involved in the immune response may be affected by noradrenergic neurotransmitters. It has been observed too that NA may be involved in the alteration of the inflammatory mechanisms in MetS [3, 20]. In healthy individuals NA generally causes falls/rises in the systemic concentrations of inflammatory/anti-inflammatory cytokines, respectively [18]. Stress system activated by the immune system stimulates a negative feedback mechanism that protects the organism from an excess of inflammatory proteins. In this way, it has been demonstrated that, in physiological situations, NA (as do catecholamines in general) inhibits the release of pro-inflammatory cytokines by Th1 lymphocytes (INF-γ, IL-2, TNF-β) but stimulates the release of anti-inflammatory cytokines by Th2 lymphocytes (IL-4, IL-10, IL-13), both of them being antagonistic responses. Similarly, catecholamines inhibit the release of other pro-inflammatory cytokines (IL-12, TNF-α) and IL-6 (a regulatory cytokine) by various immune cells and stimulate the release of the anti-inflammatory cytokines TGF-β [18]. Nonetheless, in conditions of stress and pathological inflammation, NA may induce a rise in the systemic levels of IL-6. High levels of NA and IL-6 (and IL-1β) found in obese animals may reflect defective regulation of the negative inflammatory/stress feedback loop in MetS – a physiological state that may in turn be either the cause or the consequence of diabetes associated with obesity [3]. In fact, NA can also induce the local release of TNF-α under certain pathological conditions [18], and the noradrenaline-mediated inhibition of inflammatory cytokines is altered in macrophages from obese Zucker rats: NA inhibits the IL-6 production by macrophages from lean rats but promotes IL-6 release in obese rats [20], as will be further commented.

Noradrenaline is involved as one of the first “danger or stress signals” in stress or homeostatic imbalance of the organism [21]. Danger theory assumes that the immune system may be activated by both antigenic stimuli and endogenous danger signals via the recognition of molecular schemes of danger or no danger [22]. NA is also involved in the release into the circulation of the 72 kDa extracellular heat shock protein (eHsp72) [23], which has been considered to be one of the main “danger signals” for activating the inflammatory response in several physiological stress situations, including metabolic dysregulation. Thus, Hsp72 plays an important role in physiology and human health. Under normal physiological conditions, it is expressed at low levels. However, a wide variety of pathological (including inflammation and metabolic disorders) and physiological stressful stimuli can induce a marked increase in its intracellular synthesis and extracellular release. It has been reported that intracellular Hsp72 can protect against obesity-induced IR by blocking inflammation in the context of both genetic obesity and obesity induced by high-fat feeding. In addition, a high basal concentration of extracellular Hsp72 is also associated with such disorders as hypertension, arteriosclerosis, and T2D in human and animal models. Thus, patients with T2D present low-grade inflammation, reduced gene expression of Hsp72, and elevated levels of antibody to Hsp70 (as reviewed in [24]).

In the obese Zucker rat (fa/fa, an experimental model of genetic obesity), there have also been observed, in parallel with a state of hyperglycemia and low-grade inflammation (increased levels of IL-1β, IL-6, TNF-α, and CRP), elevated circulating levels of the stress mediators NA and Hsp72 [3, 24]. The greater circulating eHsp72 concentration in these obese animals could be either a cause or a consequence of the inflammatory and stress dysregulation underlying MetS. It is thus plausible to speculate that the elevated circulating concentration of eHsp72 essentially constitutes a physiological adaptation in MetS so that the increased circulating concentration of eHsp72 in the obese animals may be actually more a consequence than a cause of MetS-related disorders [24].

It is crucial to clarify whether the underlying inflammation in MetS is the cause or the consequence of this dysregulation in stress biomarkers. It is therefore very important to resolve the controversy surrounding the effects of IL-6, whether inflammatory (pro- or anti-) or endocrine (inducing or not inducing IR, and therefore hypo- or hyperglycemic). This apparent dysregulation of the "inflammation/stress" negative feedback loop reflects a physiological situation that may in turn be either the cause or the consequence of obesity-related diabetes and therefore increase the likelihood of developing a cardiovascular disease. Considering together the systemic levels of inflammatory and stress markers in obese animals, it is plausible to hypothesize that raised circulating levels of IL-6 may be at the origin (and a good marker) of metabolic and "neuroendocrine/stress" inflammatory dysregulation in MetS. Thus, the elevation of IL-6 would induce increased systemic release of NA (which in turn would induce the elevation of eHsp72), whose high level (together with TNF-α) would be involved in the hyperglycemia also detected in these animals. Elevated levels of IL-6 would also induce an increased release of CRP, demonstrating the pro inflammatory state in MetS. In a context of deregulated stress/inflammation negative feedback system, high systemic levels of NA could stimulate (or at least not inhibit) the release of IL-6 and contribute to increasing blood levels of glucose (Fig. 3.1).

Local Inflammatory Activity and Its Dysregulation in Response to Stress Mediators

The systemic dysregulation between inflammatory and stress biomarkers in MetS may be just a consequence of the altered inflammatory and stress responses locally. A local inflammation is observed in the adipose tissue, liver, and skeletal muscle in

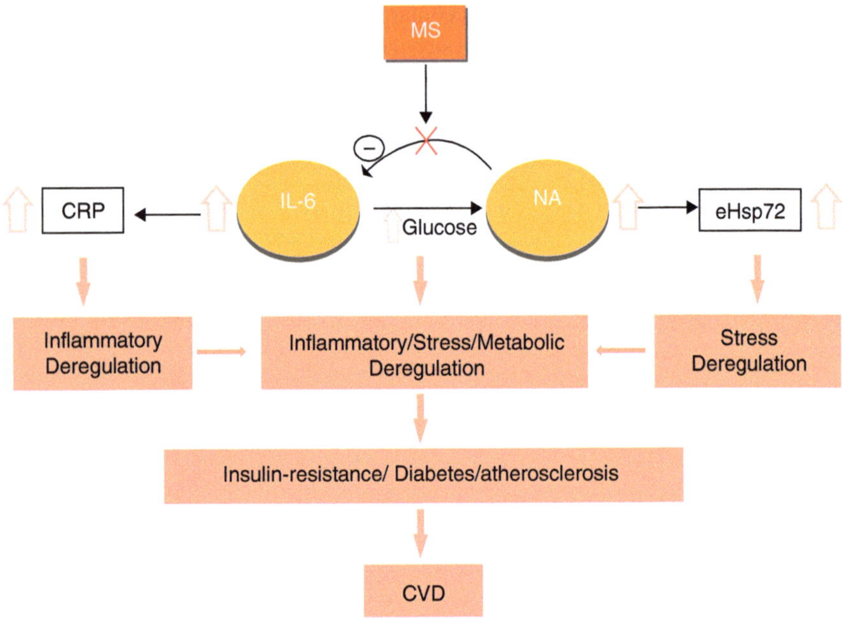

Fig. 3.1 Hypothesis of dysregulated inflammatory/stress/metabolic interaction mechanisms in metabolic syndrome. *MS* metabolic syndrome, *CRP* C-reactive protein, *IL-6* interleukin-6, *NA* noradrenaline, *eHsp72* 72 kDa extracellular heat shock protein

the pathogenesis of MetS and T2D, but its role in obesity-related metabolic disorders remains to be well determined [7]. It has been increasingly recognized that an imbalance of pro-inflammatory and anti-inflammatory adipokines contributes to the development of obesity-linked disorders. Dysregulation of anti-inflammatory adipokines caused by fat accumulation also participates in local or systemic inflammatory responses, thereby leading to the initiation or progression of metabolic and CVD [25]. Thus, there has been described a dysregulation in the synthesis and release of adipocytokines by adipocytes or by infiltrated macrophages in the adipose tissue of obese subjects: elevated secretion of the pro-inflammatory adipocytokines (TNF-α, IL-6, haptoglobin, leptin, resistin) and reduced secretion of the anti-inflammatory ones (adiponectin). Infiltration of macrophages into tissues is an important source of circulating inflammatory molecules [26]. These pro-inflammatory cytokines (including TNF-α, IL-6, and IL-1β) produced by infiltrated macrophages act in an autocrine and paracrine manner to promote IR by interfering with insulin signaling in peripheral tissues through activation of the c-JUN N-terminal kinase (JNK) and nuclear factor-kappa B (NF-kB) pathways [27]. Therefore, adipose tissue appears to play a central role in the induction of inflammation, and over-nutrition leads to changes in its cellular composition and production of pro-inflammatory cytokines and chemokines [7].

As reviewed by Esser and coworkers [7], macrophages can be classified into two distinct subtypes: the "classically activated macrophages," a pro-inflammatory phenotype termed M1 macrophages which release pro-inflammatory cytokines such as IL-1β, IL-6, TNF-α, and nitric oxide (NO), and the "alternatively activated macrophages," an anti-inflammatory phenotype termed M2 macrophages which release anti-inflammatory cytokines such as IL-10 [28]. While well established in mice [29, 30], the existence of M1 and M2 macrophage subsets has not been confirmed in human adipose tissue, where macrophages seem to be a mix of the M1 and M2 phenotypes [31]. Nonobese, physically active, and healthy dieted people maintain an "anti-inflammatory phenotype of adipose tissue" (small adipocyte size and the presence of M2 macrophages). Increased visceral fat induced by a positive energy balance and physical inactivity provokes "inflamed adipose tissue" characterized by predominant infiltrated M1 macrophages [32]. In addition, obesity can cause a phenotypic switch from the M2 to M1 phenotype, correlating with IR in both mice and humans [29–31]. Direct and paracrine signals issued from M1 macrophages can impair insulin signaling and adipogenesis in adipocytes, whereas M2 macrophages seem to protect against obesity-induced IR [28]. In addition, there is evidence that both TLR2 and TLR4 (toll-like receptors involved in the innate and inflammatory responses of immune cells, particularly macrophages) can recognize fatty acids that contribute to the release of pro-inflammatory cytokines by macrophages [33].

In obese Zucker rats, it has also been observed that peritoneal macrophages (not infiltrated in adipose tissue) exhibit a local dysregulation with respect to the constitutive or spontaneous release of pro-inflammatory cytokines, which could also be contributing to the low-grade systemic pro-inflammatory state in MetS and thus affecting the development of CVD [3, 34].

Also, the peritoneal macrophages not infiltrated in the adipose tissue show impaired release of such pro-inflammatory cytokines as IL-1β, INF-γ [34], IL-6, and TNF-α [3] in response to an antigen (lipopolysaccharide) stimulus, thus potentially increasing susceptibility to infection. This functional defect may be one of the causes of the increased susceptibility to candidiasis observed in obese individuals [35]. Indeed, the increased candidicide activity of macrophages of the obese animals could be considered to be an adaptation to this phenomenon [36]. As indicated previously, these cells also exhibit altered release of inflammatory cytokines in response to "stress messengers" or "endogenous danger signals" such as NA and Hsp72, even to animals with MetS changing their stimulatory or inhibitory effects on the release of inflammatory cytokines, particularly of IL-6 and IL-1β [20, 24]. It is therefore plausible to conclude that, in addition to systemic dysregulation in MetS, there appears local dysregulation of the innate and inflammatory responses, which not only involves infiltrated macrophages but also non-infiltrated macrophages such as the peritoneal macrophages as is manifested both in fewer of these cells in the peritoneal exudate (which may be due to increased infiltration in adipose tissue) and in impaired functional capacity [3, 20, 24, 34]. All of this serves to confirm the altered innate and inflammatory immune response capacity mediated by macrophages in MetS, corroborating the hypothesis of dysregulation in the neuroendocrine-immune response that can arise in this pathology.

Altered Response to Exercise-Induced Stress in the Metabolic Syndrome

It is now clear that obesity, T2D, and CVD share an environment characterized by IR and inflammation [27]. Therefore, removal of the inflammatory mediator signals is a more than promising strategy for the management of MetS. The potential anti-inflammatory effects of exercise have been strongly proposed as being an essential exercise-induced mechanism for improving diabetic status and insulin sensitivity by controlling the low-grade systemic inflammation associated with MetS [4, 32, 34, 37]. It has been explained above, as proposed by Gleeson and coworkers, that while a healthy diet together with exercise maintains the anti-inflammatory phenotype of adipose tissue (with predominant M2 anti-inflammatory macrophages), inactivity and an excess of energy balance lead to pro-inflammatory M1 macrophages predominating in the "inflamed adipose tissue." In this way, regular exercise decreases the risk of chronic metabolic and CVD in part because exercise exerts anti-inflammatory effects that may be mediated by both a reduction in the visceral fat mass and the induction of an anti-inflammatory environment [32]. In addition, exercise training not only inhibits inflammation in adipose tissue via suppression of macrophage infiltration but also through a phenotypic switch from M1 to M2 macrophages [38].

Nevertheless, it is clearly accepted that exercise is a form of stress and that the relation between exercise, stress, and inflammation is a good model of neuroendocrine interactions. Exercise stimulates the innate immune responses, and its effects on the inflammatory response are primarily mediated through the hypothalamic-pituitary-adrenal (HPA) axis and the SNS. A well-controlled and regulated stimulation of the innate and/or inflammatory mechanisms during exercise can help to prevent infection, but over-stimulation of the inflammatory response could also be harmful for people with inflammatory diseases, as it is the case in MetS and cardiovascular-associated disorders [3]. Thus, the anti-inflammatory hypothesis of exercise and its physiological implications needs to be clarified, particularly in the management of pathologies with inflammatory dysregulation, such as MetS. Today, it is still not formally proven whether or not an induced anti-inflammatory effect of exercise in healthy people (with an optimal neuroendocrine and inflammatory feedback) is good for the optimal regulation of homeostasis. The anti-inflammatory effects of exercise should be mainly (or only) beneficial for people with an unhealthily high inflammatory status. Further studies to define the duration and intensities of exercise programs that restore anti-inflammatory responses and the optimal cytokine-HPA axis feedback circuit, avoiding unhealthy pro-inflammatory and stress responses, are clearly necessary. For example, an inappropriate intensity of regular exercise performed by animals with MetS presenting a dysregulation in the inflammatory/stress feedback mechanisms (mediated by IL-6 and NA) can worsen this dysregulation still more by increasing circulating levels of NA, IL-6, and glucose [3] and by increasing the tissue expression and circulating levels of TNF-α, all together with a higher innate (phagocytic and microbicidal capacity) response of peritoneal macrophages [3]. These effects seem to reflect that intense regular exercise, while inducing a greater protection against infection, could exacerbate some aspects of inflammatory conditions, and intensity and duration of exercise inducing anti-inflammatory effects could compromise the immune system against pathogen challenges.

Altered response to exercise-induced stress in MetS is also manifest after single bouts of exercise. Thus, the regulation by exercise of the altered inflammatory and stress status in MetS depends on the basal set point of each individual, being anti-inflammatory mainly (or only) during a high inflammatory status. Thus, acute exercise only decreased the systemic level of IL-6, NA (also dopamine), and glucose in obese rats with the highest basal levels of these biomarkers [3].

In sum, it seems that both the pro-inflammatory and the anti-inflammatory effects of exercise may cause an additional cost (side effect) in chronic low-grade inflammatory diseases such as MetS, exacerbating the inflammatory condition (if pro-inflammatory) or increasing the susceptibility to infections (if anti-inflammatory). A good "bioregulation" of adequate intensities and durations of exercise needs to achieve a decrease in unhealthy inflammatory biomarkers together with optimal phagocytic and microbicidal activities, and clearly further studies are needed in this direction.

Molecular Mechanisms Implicated in Cardiometabolic Risk

The aim of this section is to highlight prominent molecular signals and pathways in T2D that have been linked to the development of cardiovascular disease in humans. A particular emphasis is placed on processes that have been implicated in both the pathogenesis of diabetes itself and its vascular and cardiac complications, since it is increasingly clear that these conditions often coexist as a pathologic continuum collectively referred to as "cardiometabolic disease." This chapter section is arranged into three essential parts: (1) circulating factors that have been linked to the development of diabetes and cardiovascular disease, (2) prominent molecular mechanisms that lead to vascular dysfunction and disease in diabetes, and (3) links between diabetes and the development of cardiomyopathy (heart failure).

Circulating Markers of Cardiovascular Disease in Diabetes

This part highlights three major biomarkers of diabetes that are both predictive of cardiovascular complications in epidemiological studies and mechanistically linked to the pathogenesis of diabetes and cardiovascular disease in basic and/or clinical studies.

Glucose Homeostasis Disruption

Diabetes mellitus encompasses multiple pathologies with distinct etiologies. Type 1 diabetes (T1D) is an autoimmune disease that results from a loss of pancreatic β-cells, thereby eliminating insulin production and systemic response to hyperglycemia. T2D is characterized in its early stage by impaired uptake of glucose by peripheral tissues in response to insulin, a phenomenon known as IR. Pancreatic β-cells are initially able to compensate for the resulting hyperglycemia by increasing insulin production and secretion, but this results in progressive cell hypertrophy and stress that ultimately leads to β-cell loss. Thus, the late stage of type 2 disease resembles T1D. Overall, diabetes mellitus is characterized by the inability to maintain glucose homeostasis with the consequent extended periods of hyperglycemia and also the dangerous appearance of hypoglycemia episodes.

Multiple epidemiological studies indicate that diabetic patients have an increased incidence of cardiovascular diseases compared with nondiabetic subjects. Extended daily periods of hyperglycemia are a major reason for this elevated cardiovascular risk [39]. Chronic and postprandial hyperglycemia promotes biochemical reactions leading to the glycation of proteins, lipids, or nucleic acids in peripheral tissues, generating a variety of compounds collectively known as advanced glycation end products (AGEs). The kidney is the major organ responsible for AGE clearance, which could explain the association of increased levels of circulating AGEs with renal dysfunction in diabetics. AGEs can act extracellularly or bind to receptors that signal intracellularly, such us AGEs receptor (RAGEs), to trigger several pathogenic effects on the vasculature and heart discussed further in subsequent sections.

It is important to mention that in addition to hyperglycemia, it has been shown that glucose fluctuations (hyperglycemic peaks and hypoglycemic valleys) trigger inflammatory responses and oxidative stress leading to vascular endothelial dysfunction and increased cardiovascular risk [40]. Therefore, a full understanding of the pathogenic effects elicited by poor glucose control requires well-controlled clinical studies employing continuous glucose measurement systems addressing glucose variability in the development of vascular complications.

Adipokine Imbalance

Obesity accounts for more than 80 % of the risk of developing T2D. Physical inactivity and an increased energy intake due to a diet rich in simple carbohydrates and saturated fat are related to the growing incidence of overweight and obesity around the world. The World Health Organization reported that in 2008 more than 1.4 billion adults were either overweight or already obese. Obesity is characterized by excessive fat accumulation in adipose tissue as well as ectopic lipid accumulation in organs such us liver, skeletal muscle, and cardiac muscle. Adipose tissue is not only the major tissue for lipid storage but also plays a critical role as an endocrine organ. The peptide hormones secreted by adipose tissue are known as adipokines or adipocytokines. In the last decades a growing number of studies demonstrated a clear relationship between adipokine levels and cardiovascular complications [41]. Pro-inflammatory cytokines have been discussed in a previous section of this chapter, therefore discussion will be limited specifically to the effects of adipokines.

Adipokine production and secretion responds to changes in adipose tissue mass, stress, and inflammatory states that could, through multiple mechanisms, influence cardiovascular disease risk. Leptin was the first adipokine discovered in 1994. This hormone is a major regulator of energy balance by direct actions on hypothalamic neurons that regulate food intake and energy expenditure. Circulating leptin levels are directly correlated with adipose tissue mass. Thus, obesity-related T2D is characterized by hyperleptinemia and leptin resistance. It has been reported that chronic hyperleptinemia may promote atherosclerosis by stimulating monocyte migration, increasing production of reactive oxygen species (ROS) in endothelial cells, and promoting vascular inflammation and thrombosis [42]. Therefore, interventions aimed at reducing circulating leptin levels and/or improving leptin sensitivity could have a positive impact on cardiovascular risk. Indeed, lowering circulating leptin levels may be one of the positive effects of weight loss after gastric bypass surgery.

Adiponectin is another adipokine primarily expressed and secreted by mature adipocytes. Its main functions are the stimulation of fatty acid oxidation and reduction of hepatic gluconeogenesis and plasma glucose levels. In contrast to leptin, adiponectin has anti-inflammatory and anti-atherogenic properties. Unfortunately, circulating adiponectin levels are significantly reduced in obesity-related T2D, which may result from elevations of pro-inflammatory cytokines, such as TNF-α, known to suppress adipocyte adiponectin expression. Thus, interventions that increase plasma levels of adiponectin could be beneficial to prevent cardiovascular risk or ameliorate cardiovascular complications. For example, adipose tissue reduction by bariatric surgery leads to increased levels of circulating adiponectin and potently reduces cardiovascular risk [43]. Drug treatments such as peroxisome proliferator-activated receptor gamma (PPAR-γ) agonists (e.g., pioglitazone) and angiotensin-converting enzyme inhibitors have also been successful raising circulating adiponectin levels, with well-known cardioprotective effects.

Other adipokines have also been studied, but less extensively, to assess their potential role in cardiovascular disease; this is the case of resistin and omentin-1. Circulating levels of resistin are elevated in obese and T2D subjects. Resistin is not secreted by adipocytes but is expressed in macrophages, which could explain its role in inflammation. Regarding cardiovascular risk, resistin has been related to the development of endothelial dysfunction, thrombosis, angiogenesis, and smooth muscle dysfunction [44]. Omentin-1 elicits anti-inflammatory and insulin-sensitizing effects, while also promoting vasodilation, but in a similar manner to adiponectin, omentin-1 expression is downregulated in obesity and T2D [45].

Diabetic Dyslipidemia

While the damaging effect of hyperglycemia on the cardiovascular system is well established, improving glucose control only modestly reduces cardiovascular risk in diabetic populations [46]. It is becoming increasingly recognized that aggressive management of diabetic dyslipidemia is also of critical importance. Chronic elevations in circulating free fatty acids in obesity/diabetes increase hepatic production and release of triglyceride-rich VLDL. This promotes a characteristic lipid “triad” of elevated serum triglycerides, small-dense low-density lipoprotein cholesterol (sdLDL-C), and reduced HDL-C, often with no change in total LDL [47]. Elevations of circulating free fatty acids are also implicated in the pathogenesis of IR; thus targeting this early lipid abnormality (e.g., with fibrates or thiazolidinediones) may substantially reduce cardiometabolic risk in patients with diabetes and MetS.

Mechanistic Links Between Diabetes and Vascular Dysfunction

Following the general order of topics from the previous section, a summary of the mechanistic roles of these biomarker/systems in the pathogenesis of vascular dysfunction/disease in diabetics is detailed.

Hyperglycemia Increases Production of Reactive Oxygen Species and Advanced Glycation End Products

As already mentioned, the uncontrolled and extended daily periods of hyperglycemia characteristic of diabetes are mediators of the increased cardiovascular risk observed in diabetic patients. Regarding vascular complications, endothelial dysfunction is an early event in the etiology of diabetes that leads to atherosclerosis in the long term. Hyperglycemia leads to mitochondrial dysfunction and increased ROS production in endothelial cells, compounded by elevated flux through the pentose phosphate pathway (exacerbating ROS production) and the formation of AGEs. The increase in ROS impairs angiogenesis and induces a metabolic switch reducing glycolysis and activating fatty acid oxidation, both of which may lead to vascular dysfunction. AGEs alter the extracellular matrix leading to vascular complications. AGEs act intracellularly through the activation of the receptor for AGEs to promote vascular inflammation and activate signaling cascades that reduce NO production and increase ROS production mediated by nicotinamide adenine dinucleotide phosphate (NADPH) oxidase [48]. AGEs also activate mitogen-activated protein kinases (MAPK), which along with ROS are able to activate the nuclear transcription factor NF-κB, which triggers the transcription of several pro-inflammatory cytokines, intracellular adhesion molecules, and the vascular endothelial growth factor (VEGF) [49]. Hyperglycemia also impairs the ability of endothelial nitric oxide synthase (eNOS) to produce nitric oxide (NO) by depleting arginine (substrate needed for the

NO formation), which "uncouples" the enzyme leading to superoxide production. This further reduces NO bioavailability and increases production of peroxynitrite, which elicits toxic effects by oxidizing and nitrosylating cellular proteins such as those involved in oxidative phosphorylation in mitochondria, further promoting endothelial dysfunction.

Imbalance of Adipokine Signals

As mentioned above, obesity-related T2D patients are characterized by high levels of circulating leptin. Hyperleptinemia has been identified as an independent risk factor, mediating endothelial dysfunction and neointimal hyperplasia leading to atherosclerotic coronary artery disease and arterial hypertension [42]. The molecular mechanisms implicated in leptin actions at the cellular level are mediated through different leptin receptors. Leptin receptor signaling interacts with several different signaling pathways, mainly Janus kinase/signal transducers and activators of transcription (JAK/STAT) and adenosine monophosphate-activated protein kinase (AMPK) pathways, but can also mediate its signaling through the MAPK and PI3K-Akt pathways. Leptin action is inhibited by cytokine signaling 3 receptors (SOCS3). Through its action on PI3K-Akt and MAPK, leptin influences vascular tone and promotes endothelial and smooth vascular muscle proliferation and migration. Chronic hyperleptinemia also increases ROS production and decreases NO levels in endothelial cells, leading to vascular endothelial dysfunction. This effect is compounded by leptin-induced upregulation of endothelin-1, a potent vasoconstrictor, along with multiple mediators of vascular inflammation such as TNF-α, monocyte chemotactic protein-1 (MCP-1), IL-2, and IL-6 from endothelial cells and peripheral blood mononuclear cells, increasing risk of atherogenesis.

Adiponectin elicits anti-inflammatory and anti-atherogenic properties by multiple mechanisms of action that are lost in obesity/IR and may contribute to the development of diabetes and its cardiovascular complications [50, 51]. Perivascular adipose tissue senses β-adrenergic signaling that activates eNOS and NO production, which through its actions on mitochondria triggers adiponectin release into the circulation. Adiponectin binds to collagen, allowing it to accumulate in the subendothelial space of vascular walls where it represses the expression of adhesion molecules such as the intracellular adhesion molecule-1 (ICAM-1), vascular cell AM-1 (VCAM-1), and endothelial-selectin by inhibiting TNF-α and NF-kB. This minimizes monocyte attachment to endothelial cells and polarizes resident macrophages toward the anti-inflammatory M2 phenotype, thereby reducing foam cell formation by reducing cholesterol ester accumulation. Adiponectin also promotes endothelium-dependent vasodilation by binding adiponectin receptor 1 present in smooth muscle and endothelial cells, where it triggers NO formation and release through AMPK activation. NO in smooth muscle activates cyclic guanosine monophosphate (cGMP)-dependent protein kinase events that reduce intracellular Ca^{2+} levels (e.g., by opening of large calcium-sensitive potassium channels), leading to smooth muscle relaxation and vasodilation. Obesity/IR inhibits these vasculoprotective processes by blocking adiponectin signaling, impairing β-adrenergic receptor sensitivity, and reducing adiponectin and AMPK expression. As a consequence, blood vessels are vasoconstricted and more atherogenic, which compounded by hyperglycemia and dyslipidemia potentially increases cardiovascular risk.

Dyslipidemia and Vascular Disease in Diabetes

While hyperglycemia and adipokine imbalance clearly contribute to the pathogenesis of vascular disease in diabetics, lipid abnormalities such as decreased serum HDL-C, elevated sdLDL-C, and hypertriglyceridemia are believed to be of primary importance in precipitating coronary artery disease in diabetics [47]. Visceral adiposity, IR, and enhanced SNS activity associated with the MetS result in a chronic elevation of serum free fatty acids, which enhances hepatic VLDL-C and triglyceride (TG) synthesis and secretion. Prolonged elevation of VLDL and TGs, particularly postprandially due to IR, promotes sdLDL-C production in diabetics by enriching LDL particles and TGs that are subsequently modified by hepatic lipase and cholesterol ester transfer protein [52]. sdLDL-C is more susceptible to oxidation and adhesion to the vascular endothelium than LDL-C, making it particularly atherogenic and highly predictive of vascular endothelial dysfunction in diabetics [53]. Elevated TGs and hepatic lipase activity also modify the size, composition, and catabolic rate of HDL-C, ultimately reducing levels of this anti-atherogenic lipoprotein. Obesity/IR alters several other enzymes and regulatory pathways involved in hepatic and intestinal lipoprotein synthesis and release that are beyond the scope of this chapter (see [54] for review), which combine to make the mechanisms of dyslipidemia in diabetes particularly complex. Figure 3.2 presents an overview of the aforementioned mechanisms.

Diabetic Cardiomyopathy

IR and MetS are independent risk factors for heart failure, and diabetes patients are up to five times more likely to have heart failure than the general population. In addition to the well-established pathogenic effects of hyperglycemia and hyperlipidemia on the coronary vasculature, diabetes and MetS are associated with a distinct form of cardiac dysfunction known as "diabetic cardiomyopathy" (DMCM) that occurs independent of the precipitating effects of coronary artery disease, hyperlipidemia, or arterial hypertension [55]. The etiology of this condition involves the complex interaction of metabolic, neurohormonal, and subcellular derangements that directly affect myocardial cells prior to the onset of overt diabetes or cardiac dysfunction. This section of the chapter will summarize the accumulating evidence from basic, translational, and clinical studies for the distinct effects of diabetes and MetS on the heart that support to the increasing consensus that novel therapeutic approaches may be needed to prevent and optimally manage heart failure in this patient population.

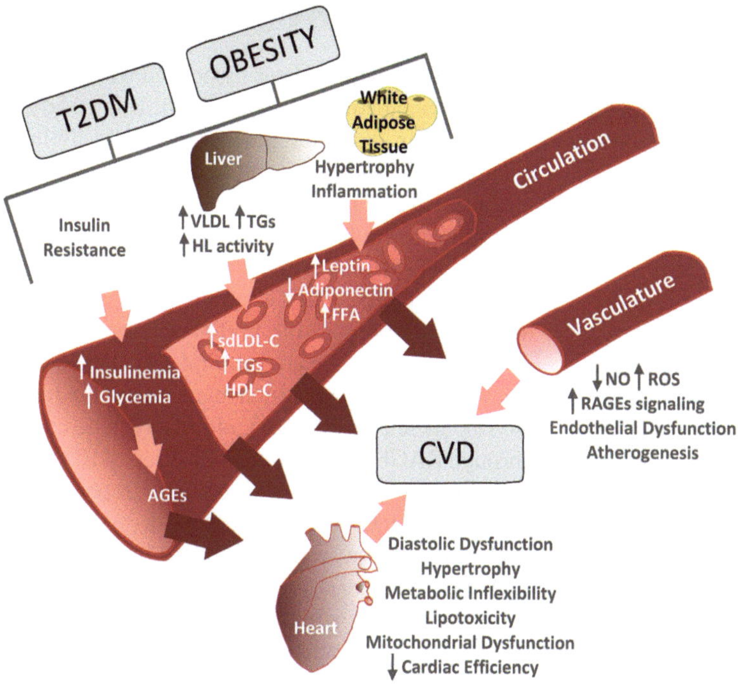

Fig. 3.2 Overview of the mechanisms and players involved in type 2 diabetes-related cardiovascular disorders. *T2DM* type 2 diabetes mellitus, *VLDL* very low-density lipoprotein, *TGs* triglycerides, *FFA* free fatty acids, *sdLDL-C* small-dense low-density lipoprotein cholesterol, *HDL-C* high-density lipoprotein cholesterol, *AGEs* advanced glycation end products, *NO* nitric oxide, *ROS* reactive oxygen species, *RAGEs* advanced glycation end products receptor, *CVD* cardiovascular disorders

Organ Level Changes

The early stage pathology of DMCM is an increase in left ventricular (LV) wall thickness associated with interstitial accumulation of AGEs and reduced compliance [56], which later progresses to involve interstitial and perivascular fibrosis and cardiomyocyte hypertrophy. These changes contribute to an impairment of LV diastolic function, which is typically the first detectable sign of cardiac dysfunction in diabetes and MetS. Hyperglycemia is postulated to play an important role in this early fibrosis by increasing AGE formation, which promotes myocardial collagen deposition and pro-inflammatory signaling. This may be compounded by impaired myocardial energetics, lipid droplet formation (steatosis), and cardiomyocyte damage or loss due to oxidative stress and apoptosis (discussed below). Diastolic dysfunction may progress toward LV dilatation and compromised systolic function as is seen in classic heart failure pathogenesis, perhaps accelerated by alterations in myocardial metabolic substrate utilization, mitochondrial dysfunction, and reduced cardiac efficiency.

Toxic Effects of Hyperglycemia and Hyperinsulinemia

Hyperglycemia is a hallmark of diabetes and has been associated with elevated heart failure risk in both diabetic and nondiabetic populations [57]. It is widely considered to be a central initiating factor in the development of DMCM by increasing cardiac oxidative stress, inflammation, and maladaptive remodeling by activating pathogenic signaling by the myocardial renin-angiotensin system, transforming growth factor (TGF)-β/insulin-like growth factor 1 (IGF-1) (via hyperinsulinemia), and poly(ADP ribose) polymerase (PARP). A primary mediator of glucose toxicity in the heart is likely the formation of AGEs, which accumulate in tissues of diabetic patients and are thought to play an important role in diabetic complications. The precise chemistry and cellular actions of AGEs are incompletely understood, but it is generally accepted that their formation begins by nonenzymatic binding of glucose to amino acids or deoxyribonucleic acid (DNA), ultimately generating a variety of compounds that act through RAGEs to promote production of ROS, crosslink collagen, and induce pro-inflammatory (e.g., NF-κB) and hypertrophic (e.g., extracellular signal-regulated kinases [ERK]/MAPK) signaling [49].

A common pathogenic link among these systems activated by hyperglycemia is thought to be the generation of ROS by a variety of sources including NADPH oxidase, uncoupled eNOS, and mitochondria, perhaps compounded reduced cardiac antioxidant enzyme capacity. The ensuing oxidative and nitrosative stress can damage cellular proteins and lipids, leading to impairments in Ca^{2+} homeostasis, myocardial impulse conduction, and microvascular function [58]. Adding further insult to injury, hyperglycemia, in part by inducing hyperinsulinemia, also impairs cardiac autophagy by inhibition of AMPK and activation of mammalian target of rapamycin (mTOR) signaling, resulting in an aggregation of damaged proteins and cellular components in the diabetic heart [59]. This loss of cellular "quality control" has been linked to endoplasmic reticulum (ER) stress and mitochondrial dysfunction, further contributing to myocardial dysfunction and disease progression.

Cardiac Lipotoxicity and Altered Myocardial Energy Metabolism

In addition to the toxic effects of hyperglycemia on the myocardium, diabetes also alters myocardial energy metabolism by influencing the partitioning of metabolic substrates and inducing mitochondrial dysfunction [60–62]. Under normal conditions, the heart relies primarily on fatty acid oxidation to support energy requirements, which fuels aerobic adenosine triphosphate (ATP) production by mitochondrial oxidative phosphorylation. However, the heart is often referred to as a "metabolic omnivore," capable of switching substrate utilization to glucose, lactate, ketones, or amino acids given changes in metabolic demand or substrate availability [63]. In the diabetic heart, this metabolic flexibility is lost, due to cardiac IR and glucose transporter type 4 (GLUT-4) downregulation, compounded by an oversupply of fatty acids that allosterically inhibit glucose oxidation and transcriptionally upregulates fatty acid transport and oxidation via activation of PPAR-α/PPAR-γ coactivator 1 (PGC-1) signaling network. However, this enhanced uptake of fatty acids by cardiomyocytes appears to exceed mitochondrial capacity to oxidize them, leading to a cellular accumulation of nonesterified fatty acids, triglycerides, and toxic lipid intermediates such as ceramides. This may lead to myocardial steatosis and "cardiac lipotoxicity," which are thought to play an important role in DMCM remodeling by exacerbating cardiac IR and promoting cardiomyocyte apoptosis, ER stress, inflammation, and mitochondrial dysfunction [64].

Interestingly, elevated use of lipid by the diabetic heart is also associated with increased myocardial oxygen consumption for a given amount of work in animal models [65]. This apparent reduction in cardiac efficiency may compound metabolic inflexibility during times of metabolic stress, such as ischemia, rendering the heart unable to adequately meet energy demands and therefore more susceptible to injury and arrhythmogenesis. The loss of myocardial efficiency may involve an uncoupling of mitochondrial respiration from oxidative phosphorylation in cardiomyocytes, perhaps due to enhanced expression and activities of uncoupling proteins and/or the adenine nucleotide translocase [65, 66]. Dissipation of mitochondrial membrane potential by these mechanisms likely serves to initially limit mitochondrial ROS formation but at the expense of ATP generation, which may ultimately contribute to the progressive metabolic stress and remodeling in the diabetic heart. Indeed, reductions in myocardial phosphocreatine/ATP ratios, measured by phosphorus 31-nuclear magnetic resonance (^{31}P-NMR) spectroscopy in vivo, have been reported in diabetic patients with both normal and impaired cardiac function by echocardiography [67].

Inflammation as a Therapeutic Target in Diabetes Mellitus: A Clinical View

In recent years, the role of the immune system in the pathophysiology of diabetes has been reconsidered, and different approaches have been made public. If, on one hand, its role in the origin of T1D is indisputable, it is not as evident in relation to T2D, the focus of this section. However, it seems logical to assume that if the immune system has the function to respond to pathogens and to mechanical or chemical insults, it should also be able to react against an excess of nutrients, aiming to restore homeostasis.

In fact, several lines of evidence published over the last years have the merit of clearly demonstrating the relationship between obesity (with its associated metabolic stress) and inflammation. Specifically in T2D patients, several papers had come to call attention to increased serum levels of typical inflammation biomarkers, such as CRP, cortisol, sialic acid, α-1 acid glycoprotein, serum amyloid A, and proinflammatory cytokines, like IL-6 [68–71]. Further, TNF-α was found to play an active role in the development of IR [72], and IL-1β was implicated in insulin secretion defects [73], along with similar observations connecting inflammatory mediators with some complications of T2D, such as cardiovascular and renal diseases [74, 75]. Cells of the immune system have also been implicated in pathophysiological mechanisms, and some proof-of-concept clinical studies have been published, leading to the view that T2D may actually be an inflammatory disease (or, better saying, an autoinflammatory disease), being the prototype of a whole new field of research related to the new concept of immunometabolism, as was previously highlighted.

Many of these ideas are still under investigation, and, of course, they are not currently taken into consideration regarding decision-making processes, in day-to-day clinical practice. However, they represent an excellent opportunity for the development of new therapeutic strategies that, at least in the long term, may contribute to reduce T2D burden in modern societies.

Treating Type 2 Diabetes Through Inflammation Control

After identifying some inflammatory mechanisms by which pancreatic β-cells undergo damage in T2D, it is reasonable to think that inflammation itself can be a cause of the disease and, in this sense, can be a target for a causative therapy. The treatment of other diseases of inflammatory nature (such as the classical rheumatic autoimmune diseases) has been advancing in an extraordinary way, and several drugs have been developed with the aim of modulating the activity of TNF-α, IL-1α, IL-1β, and NF-κB. All these pharmacological premises have led to a rapid translation of this knowledge to clinical trials, probably (and at least initially) with unrealistic high expectations regarding T2D patients' metabolic control.

Indeed, after having discovered the role that TNF-α may have in insulin resistance [72], several clinical studies were conducted to test the hypothesis of using an anti-TNF-α drug as an active agent promoting metabolic control in T2D patients, trying to confirm some interesting preclinical data already available. However, those studies failed to confirm that hypothesis [76–81]. It is worth to say, nevertheless, that all of them suffered from some methodological issues that, in a posterior analysis, may help to understand the results: the duration of the treatment was always short (ranging from 2 days to 4 weeks), and small sample sizes were used (the number of recruited subjects ranged from 7 to 54). Thus, these trials were naturally underpowered to observe differences between populations of patients diagnosed with a very heterogeneous disease, such as T2D. Taking this into account, more recently, new studies were designed and conducted in obese patients treated with anti-TNF-α drugs, showing that blocking cytokine resulted in insulin sensitivity alterations and improvement of glycemic parameters [82–85]. Overall, these apparent contradictory results emphasize the need for a thorough clinical study, with the statistical power needed to clearly define what is actually the effect of anti-TNF-α drugs in T2D patients.

A different approach may also be considered when thinking about inflammation modulation and metabolic control in T2D: IL-1 [86–90] and NF-κB [91–94] antagonism (while seemingly two distinct pathways, the truth is that IL-1 activates

NF-κB). Using the IL-1 receptor antagonist IL-1Ra and salsalate (an anti-inflammatory drug belonging to the family of salicylates), several studies were conducted and confirmed the capacity of these pharmacological interventions to improve insulin secretion in diabetic and prediabetic patients, as well as to ameliorate the sensitivity to the same hormone in that populations, along with a decrease in blood levels of HbA1c [86–94]. It must be emphasized that IL-1 antagonism demonstrated to be mainly effective on insulin secretion, while salsalate proved to act fundamentally on insulin-sensitive tissues. In this context, it would be logical to think that a combined approach may have stronger effects, but this needs to be further investigated. In addition, some authors had also demonstrated that IL-1β might induce a prolonged hypoglycemia in mice, not caused by a reduction in food intake and being dissociable from insulin effects [95]. The biologic significance of this pathway is uncertain, but it reinforces the need for further research in this area, especially considering the possibility for therapeutic intervention in clinical practice.

Of note, most of the studies cited were performed in addition to standard therapies, and, therefore, caution should be taken when interpreting the data, since several drugs used in T2D care may have anti-inflammatory effects, like statins, acetylsalicylic acid, angiotensin-converting enzyme inhibitors, and angiotensin receptor blockers. Even classical antidiabetic drugs (such as metformin and sulfonylureas) and newer molecules (like dipeptidyl peptidase 4 inhibitors) can effectively reduce IL-1β activity [96]. This pharmacological profile may actually lead to an underestimation of the relevance of inflammation in T2D [97].

Peripheral tissue inflammation is also important in diabetes complications so that the use of anti-inflammatory drugs may also have theoretical interest in the therapeutic approach to these clinical conditions. Indeed, a large phase III clinical trial (NCT01327846) is currently recruiting patients, aiming to test the hypothesis of preventing cardiovascular disease and improving insulin secretion and glycemic parameters with subcutaneous canakinumab, an antibody directed against IL-1β. Seventeen thousand two hundred patients will be included in the study, will be submitted to treatment with different doses of the antibody every 3 months, and will be followed up over 4 years. A clinical trial of this dimension can be extremely important to assert the autoinflammatory nature of T2D-associated metabolic disorders and, thus, contribute to the effective development of a cytokine-based therapy with immediate clinical application.

The use of antibodies in T2D treatment (and particularly of its complications) is not recent. In fact, regarding the therapeutic approach of diabetic retinopathy, several molecules have frequent clinical use, particularly in association with surgical procedures. The most important drugs at this level have an anti-VEGF action. VEGF is a potent vasopermeability factor and plays an important role in the pathophysiology of diabetic retinopathy, contributing to neovascularization and alteration of the blood-retina barrier. It affects the function of endothelial tight junction proteins and leads to extravasation of fluid and retinal edema, after the breakdown of the barrier, which is also aggravated by some degree of leukostasis in the retinal microvessels [98]. Drugs that have the ability of directly blocking VEGF include the monoclonal antibody fragment ranibizumab and the full-length antibody bevacizumab. Other treatments include the anti-VEGF aptamer pegaptanib, soluble VEGF receptor analogues such as VEGF-Trap, small interfering RNAs such as bevasiranib and, finally, rapamycin, but further data on these molecules is out of the scope of this review [98].

Considering only monoclonal antibodies, ranibizumab is a fragment (Fab) that blocks all isoforms of VEGF-A. It is the only drug that has been approved for use in patients diagnosed with diabetic macular edema, and, in a study aiming to measure the impact of the drug in that clinical condition, a beneficial effect of ranibizumab in slowing down the progression of diabetic retinopathy and in improving the severity of that microvascular complication was also noted [99]. In fact, the Diabetic Retinopathy Clinical Research Network, a multicenter, randomized clinical trial showed that intravitreal administration of ranibizumab with prompt or deferred laser was more effective than prompt laser alone for up to at least 1 year, in patients with diabetic macular edema [100]. This helped to position anti-VEGF agents as first-line treatment of center-involving diabetic macular edema, and laser may be further added in refractory cases or in those with poor response to pharmacological therapy alone. Bevacizumab is a full-length humanized antibody that also blocks all isoforms of VEGF-A. Despite the absence of a formal indication, it has been used as an off-label drug for the treatment of retinal vascular diseases, such as proliferative diabetic retinopathy and diabetic macular edema. In fact, in the BOLT study (which compared intravitreal bevacizumab with laser), it was possible to observe an improvement in visual acuity (of 8 letters) with bevacizumab injections, whereas patients submitted to laser therapy experienced a loss of a median of 0.5 letters [101].

These two biological agents (ranibizumab and bevacizumab) are two paradigmatic examples of the possibility of specific and directed interventions, within what clinicians know to be T2D (and its complications) pathophysiology. With advancing knowledge on the mechanisms involved in the disease, a contemporary drug development is also expected. Inflammation provides a huge field of intervention, given the amount of molecular mediators that may be involved in the genesis and perpetuation of the disease. Therefore, it is envisaged that many of the medical developments that will occur in the area of diabetes in the near future just go through the control of inflammation. The future will tell whether we will be successful, but at least some positive perspectives are now growing up for optimal control of a disease that is a heavy burden, not only from a clinical point of view but also in personal, family, and social terms.

References

1. Eckel RH, Grundy SM, Zimmet PZ. The metabolic syndrome. Lancet. 2005;365(9468):1415–28.
2. Hotamisligil GS. Inflammation and metabolic disorders. Nature. 2006;444(7121):860–7.
3. Martín-Cordero L, García JJ, Hinchado MD, Ortega E. The interleukin-6 and noradrenaline mediated inflammation-stress feedback mechanism is dysregulated in metabolic syndrome: effect of exercise. Cardiovasc Diabetol. 2011;10:42.

4. Pedersen BK. The anti-inflammatory effect of exercise: its role in diabetes and cardiovascular disease control. Essays Biochem. 2006;42:105–17.
5. Mathis D, Shoelson S. Immunometabolism; an emerging frontier. Nat Rev Immunol. 2011;11(2):81–93.
6. Koh KK, Han SH, Quon MJ. Inflammatory markers and the metabolic syndrome: insights from therapeutic interventions. J Am Coll Cardiol. 2005;46(11):1978–85.
7. Esser N, Legrand-Poels S, Piette J, Scheen AJ, Paquot N. Inflammation as a link between obesity, metabolic syndrome and type 2 diabetes. Diabetes Res Clin Pract. 2014;105(2):141–50.
8. Trayhurn P, Wood IS. Adipokines: inflammation and the pleiotropic role of white adipose tissue. Br J Nutr. 2004;92(3):347–55.
9. Wellen KE, Hotamisligil GS. Inflammation, stress, and diabetes. J Clin Invest. 2005;115(5):1111-9.
10. Hoch M, Eberle AN, Peterli R, Peters T, Seboek D, Keller U, et al. LPS induces interleukin-6 and interleukin-8 but not tumor necrosis factor-alpha in human adipocytes. Cytokine. 2008;41(1):29–37.
11. Bastard JP, Maachi M, Lagathu C, Kim MJ, Caron M, Vidal H, et al. Recent advances in the relationship between obesity, inflammation, and insulin resistance. Eur Cytokine Netw. 2006;17(1):4–12.
12. Mirza S, Hossain M, Mathews C, Martinez P, Pino P, Gay JL, et al. Type 2-diabetes is associated with elevated levels of TNF-alpha, IL-6 and adiponectin and low levels of leptin in a population of Mexican Americans: a cross-sectional study. Cytokine. 2012;57(1):136–42.
13. Eder K, Baffy N, Falus A, Fulop AK. The major inflammatory mediator interleukin-6 and obesity. Inflamm Res. 2009;58(11):727–36.
14. van Hall G, Steensberg A, Sacchetti M, Fischer C, Keller C, Schjerling P, et al. Interleukin-6 stimulates lipolysis and fat oxidation in humans. J Clin Endocrinol Metab. 2003;88(7):3005–10.
15. Timpson NJ, Lawlor DA, Harbord RM, Gaunt TR, Day IN, Palmer LJ, et al. C-reactive protein and its role in metabolic syndrome: mendelian randomisation study. Lancet. 2005;366(9501):1954–9.
16. Pischon T, Hu FB, Rexrode KM, Girman CJ, Manson JE, Rimm EB. Inflammation, the metabolic syndrome, and risk of coronary heart disease in women and men. Atherosclerosis. 2008;197(1):392–9.
17. Calle MC, Fernandez ML. Inflammation and type 2 diabetes. Diabetes Metab. 2012;38:183–91.
18. Elenkov IJ, Chrousos GP. Stress hormones, proinflammatory and anti-inflammatory cytokines, and autoimmunity. Ann N Y Acad Sci. 2002;966:290–303.
19. Straznicky NE, Lambert GW, Lambert EA. Neuroadrenergic dysfunction in obesity: an overview of the effects of weight loss. Curr Opin Lipidol. 2010;21(1):21–30.
20. Martín-Cordero L, García JJ, Ortega E. Noradrenaline-mediated inhibition of inflammatory cytokines is altered in macrophages from obese Zucker rats: effect of habitual exercise. Endocr Metab Immune Disord Drug Targets. 2013;13(3):234–9.
21. Ortega E, Giraldo E, Hinchado MD, Martín L, García JJ, De la Fuente M. Neuroimmunomodulation during exercise: role of catecholamines as "stress mediator" and/or danger signal for the innate immune response. Neuroimmunomodulation. 2007;14(3–4):206–12.
22. Matzinger P. An innate sense of danger. Semin Immunol. 1998;10(5):399–415.
23. Giraldo E, Multhoff G, Ortega E. Noradrenaline increases the expression and release of Hsp72 by human neutrophils. Brain Behav Immun. 2010;24(4):672–7.
24. Garcia JJ, Martin-Cordero L, Hinchado MD, Bote ME, Ortega E. Effects of habitual exercise on the eHsp72-induced release of inflammatory cytokines by macrophages from obese Zucker rats. Int J Sports Med. 2013;34(6):559–64.
25. Ohashi K, Shibata R, Murohara T, Ouchi N. Role of anti-inflammatory adipokines in obesity-related diseases. Trends Endocrinol Metab. 2014;25(7):348–55.
26. Weisberg SP, McCann D, Desai M, Rosenbaum M, Leibel RL, Ferrante Jr AW. Obesity is associated with macrophage accumulation in adipose tissue. J Clin Invest. 2003;112(12):1796–808.

27. Shoelson SE, Lee J, Goldfine AB. Inflammation and insulin resistance. J Clin Invest. 2006;116(7):1793–801.
28. Chawla A, Nguyen KD, Goh YP. Macrophage-mediated inflammation in metabolic disease. Nat Rev Immunol. 2011;11(11):738–44.
29. Lumeng CN, Bodzin JL, Saltiel AR. Obesity induces a phenotypic switch in adipose tissue macrophage polarization. J Clin Invest. 2007;117(1):175–84.
30. Fujisaka S, Usui I, Bukhari A, Ikutani M, Oya T, Kanatani Y, et al. Regulatory mechanisms for adipose tissue M1 and M2 macrophages in diet-induced obese mice. Diabetes. 2009;58(11):2574–82.
31. Wentworth JM, Naselli G, Brown WA, Doyle L, Phipson B, Smyth GK, et al. Pro-inflammatory CD11c+CD206+ adipose tissue macrophages are associated with insulin resistance in human obesity. Diabetes. 2010;59(7):1648–56.
32. Gleeson M, Bishop NC, Stensel DJ, Lindley MR, Mastana SS, Nimmo MA. The anti-inflammatory effects of exercise: mechanisms and implications for the prevention and treatment of disease. Nat Rev Immunol. 2011;11(9):607–15.
33. Shi H, Kokoeva MV, Inouye K, Tzameli I, Yin H, Flier JS. TLR4 links innate immunity and fatty acid-induced insulin resistance. J Clin Invest. 2006;116(11):3015–25.
34. Martin-Cordero L, Garcia JJ, Giraldo E, De la Fuente M, Manso R, Ortega E. Influence of exercise on the circulating levels and macrophage production of IL-1beta and IFNgamma affected by metabolic syndrome: an obese Zucker rat experimental animal model. Eur J Appl Physiol. 2009;107(5):535–43.
35. Plotkin BJ, Paulson D, Chelich A, Jurak D, Cole J, Kasimos J, et al. Immune responsiveness in a rat model for type II diabetes (Zucker rat, fa/fa): susceptibility to *Candida albicans* infection and leucocyte function. J Med Microbiol. 1996;44(4):277–83.
36. Martin-Cordero L, Reis F, Garcia JJ, Teixeira F, Ortega E. Effect of exercise without diet on functional capacity of peritoneal macrophages and TNF-α levels in blood and in adipose tissue in the obese Zucker rat model of the metabolic syndrome. Proc Nutr Soc. 2013;72(OCE1):E76.
37. Teixeira de Lemos E, Reis F, Baptista S, Pinto R, Sepodes B, Vala H, et al. Exercise training decreases proinflammatory profile in Zucker diabetic (type 2) fatty rats. Nutrition. 2009;25(3):330–9.
38. Kawanishi N, Yano H, Yokogawa Y, Suzuki K. Exercise training inhibits inflammation in adipose tissue via both suppression of macrophage infiltration and acceleration of phenotypic switching from M1 to M2 macrophages in high-fat-diet-induced obese mice. Exerc Immunol Rev. 2010;16:105–18.
39. Haffner SJ, Cassells H. Hyperglycemia as a cardiovascular risk factor. Am J Med. 2003;115(Suppl 8A):6S–11.
40. Monnier L, Mas E, Ginet C, Michel F, Villon L, Cristol JP, et al. Activation of oxidative stress by acute glucose fluctuations compared with sustained chronic hyperglycemia in patients with type 2 diabetes. JAMA. 2006;295(14):1681–7.
41. Funahashi T, Matsuzawa Y. Adiponectin and the cardiometabolic syndrome: an epidemiological perspective. Best Pract Res Clin Endocrinol Metab. 2014;28(1):93–106.
42. Wang H, Luo W, Eitzman DT. Leptin in thrombosis and atherosclerosis. Curr Pharm Des. 2014;20(4):641–5.
43. Herder C, Peltonen M, Svensson PA, Carstensen M, Jacobson P, Roden M, et al. Adiponectin and bariatric surgery: associations with diabetes and cardiovascular disease in the Swedish Obese Subjects Study. Diabetes Care. 2014;37(5):1401–9.
44. Abate N, Sallam HS, Rizzo M, Nikolic D, Obradovic M, Bjelogrlic P, et al. Resistin: an inflammatory cytokine. Role in cardiovascular diseases, diabetes and the metabolic syndrome. Curr Pharm Des. 2014;20(31):4961–9.
45. Greulich S, Chen WJ, Maxhera B, Rijzewijk LJ, van der Meer RW, Jonker JT, et al. Cardioprotective properties of omentin-1 in type 2 diabetes: evidence from clinical and in vitro studies. PLoS One. 2013;8(3):e59697.
46. Weiss IA, Valiquette G, Schwarcz MD. Impact of glycemic treatment choices on cardiovascular complications in type 2 diabetes. Cardiol Rev. 2009;17(4):165–75.

47. Carmena R. Type 2 diabetes, dyslipidemia, and vascular risk: rationale and evidence for correcting the lipid imbalance. Am Heart J. 2005;150(5):859–70.
48. Yamagishi S. Role of advanced glycation end products (AGEs) and receptor for AGEs (RAGE) in vascular damage in diabetes. Exp Gerontol. 2011;46(4):217–24.
49. Rojas A, Morales MA. Advanced glycation and endothelial functions: a link towards vascular complications in diabetes. Life Sci. 2004;76(7):715–30.
50. Li S, Shin HJ, Ding EL, van Dam RM. Adiponectin levels and risk of type 2 diabetes: a systematic review and meta-analysis. JAMA. 2009;302(2):179–88.
51. Kishida K, Funahashi T, Shimomura I. Molecular mechanisms of diabetes and atherosclerosis: role of adiponectin. Endocr Metab Immune Disord Drug Targets. 2012;12(2):118–31.
52. Syvanne M, Taskinen MR. Lipids and lipoproteins as coronary risk factors in non-insulin-dependent diabetes mellitus. Lancet. 1997;350 Suppl 1:SI20–3.
53. Tan KC, Ai VH, Chow WS, Chau MT, Leong L, Lam KS. Influence of low density lipoprotein (LDL) subfraction profile and LDL oxidation on endothelium-dependent and independent vasodilation in patients with type 2 diabetes. J Clin Endocrinol Metab. 1999;84(9):3212–6.
54. Adiels M, Olofsson SO, Taskinen MR, Boren J. Overproduction of very low-density lipoproteins is the hallmark of the dyslipidemia in the metabolic syndrome. Arterioscler Thromb Vasc Biol. 2008;28(7):1225–36.
55. Kannel WB, Hjortland M, Castelli WP. Role of diabetes in congestive heart failure: the Framingham study. Am J Cardiol. 1974;34(1):29–34.
56. van Heerebeek L, Hamdani N, Handoko ML, Falcao-Pires I, Musters RJ, Kupreishvili K, et al. Diastolic stiffness of the failing diabetic heart: importance of fibrosis, advanced glycation end products, and myocyte resting tension. Circulation. 2008;117(1):43–51.
57. Nichols GA, Gullion CM, Koro CE, Ephross SA, Brown JB. The incidence of congestive heart failure in type 2 diabetes: an update. Diabetes Care. 2004;27(8):1879–84.
58. Varga ZV, Giricz Z, Liaudet L, Hasko G, Ferdinandy P, Pacher P. Interplay of oxidative, nitrosative/nitrative stress, inflammation, cell death and autophagy in diabetic cardiomyopathy. Biochim Biophys Acta. 2015;1852(2):232–42.
59. Kobayashi S, Liang Q. Autophagy and mitophagy in diabetic cardiomyopathy. Biochim Biophys Acta. 2015;1852(2):252–61.
60. Duncan JG. Mitochondrial dysfunction in diabetic cardiomyopathy. Biochim Biophys Acta. 2011;1813(7):1351–9.
61. Kok BP, Brindley DN. Myocardial fatty acid metabolism and lipotoxicity in the setting of insulin resistance. Heart Fail Clin. 2012;8(4):643–61.
62. Rodrigues B, Cam MC, McNeill JH. Myocardial substrate metabolism: implications for diabetic cardiomyopathy. J Mol Cell Cardiol. 1995;27(1):169–79.
63. Lopaschuk GD, Ussher JR, Folmes CD, Jaswal JS, Stanley WC. Myocardial fatty acid metabolism in health and disease. Physiol Rev. 2010;90(1):207–58.
64. van de Weijer T, Schrauwen-Hinderling VB, Schrauwen P. Lipotoxicity in type 2 diabetic cardiomyopathy. Cardiovasc Res. 2011;92(1):10–8.
65. Boudina S, Abel ED. Mitochondrial uncoupling: a key contributor to reduced cardiac efficiency in diabetes. Physiology (Bethesda). 2006;21:250–8.
66. Boudina S, Sena S, Theobald H, Sheng X, Wright JJ, Hu XX, et al. Mitochondrial energetics in the heart in obesity-related diabetes: direct evidence for increased uncoupled respiration and activation of uncoupling proteins. Diabetes. 2007;56(10):2457–66.
67. Scheuermann-Freestone M, Madsen PL, Manners D, Blamire AM, Buckingham RE, Styles P, et al. Abnormal cardiac and skeletal muscle energy metabolism in patients with type 2 diabetes. Circulation. 2003;107(24):3040–6.
68. Spranger J, Kroke A, Möhlig M, Hoffmann K, Bergmann MM, Ristow M, et al. Inflammatory cytokines and the risk to develop type 2 diabetes: results of the prospective population-based European Prospective Investigation into Cancer and Nutrition (EPIC) – Potsdam Study. Diabetes. 2003;52(3):812–7.
69. Pradhan AD, Manson JE, Rifai N, Buring JE, Ridker PM. C-reactive protein, interleukin 6, and risk of developing type 2 diabetes mellitus. JAMA. 2001;286(3):327–34.

70. Pickup JC, Crook MA. Is type II diabetes mellitus a disease of the innate immune system? Diabetologia. 1998;41(10):1241–8.
71. Pickup JC, Mattock MB, Chusney GD, Burt D. NIDDM as a disease of the innate immune system: association of acute-phase reactants and interleukin-6 with metabolic syndrome X. Diabetologia. 1997;40(11):1286–92.
72. Hotamisligil GS, Shargill NS, Spiegelman BM. Adipose expression of tumor necrosis factor-alpha: direct role in obesity-linked insulin resistance. Science. 1993;259(5091):87–91.
73. Maedler K, Sergeev P, Ris F, Oberholzer J, Joller-Jemelka HI, Spinas GA, et al. Glucose-induced beta cell production of IL-1beta contributes to glucotoxicity in human pancreatic islets. J Clin Invest. 2002;110(6):851–60.
74. Madhumitha H, Mohan V, Deepa M, Babu S, Aravindhan V. Increased Th1 and suppressed Th2 serum cytokine levels in subjects with diabetic coronary artery disease. Cardiovasc Diabetol. 2014;13:1.
75. Navarro-González JF, Mora-Fernández C. The role of inflammatory cytokines in diabetic nephropathy. J Am Soc Nephrol. 2008;19(3):433–42.
76. Lo J, Bernstein LE, Canavan B, Torriani M, Jackson MB, Ahima RS, et al. Effects of TNF-alpha neutralization on adipocytokines and skeletal muscle adiposity in the metabolic syndrome. Am J Physiol Endocrinol Metab. 2007;293(1):E102–9.
77. Rosevinge A, Krogh-Madsen R, Baslund B, Pedersen BK. Insulin resistance in patients with rheumatoid arthritis: effect of anti-TNFalpha therapy. Scand J Rheumatol. 2007;36(2):91–6.
78. Bernstein LE, Berry J, Kim S, Canavan B, Grinspoon SK. Effects of etanercept in patients with the metabolic syndrome. Arch Intern Med. 2006;166(8):902–8.
79. Dominguez H, Storgaard H, Rask-Madsen C, Steffen Hermann T, Ihlemann N, Baunbjerg Nielsen D, et al. Metabolic and vascular effects of tumor necrosis factor-alpha blockade with etanercept in obese patients with type 2 diabetes. J Vasc Res. 2005;42(6):517–25.
80. Paquot N, Castillo MJ, Lefèbvre PJ, Scheen AJ. No increased insulin sensitivity after a single intravenous administration of a recombinant human tumor necrosis factor receptor: Fc fusion protein in obese insulin-resistant patients. J Clin Endocrinol Metab. 2000;85(3):1316–9.
81. Ofei F, Hurel S, Newkirk J, Sopwith M, Taylor R. Effects of an engineered human anti-TNF-alpha antibody (CDP571) on insulin sensitivity and glycemic control in patients with NIDDM. Diabetes. 1996;45(7):881–5.
82. Stanley TL, Zanni MV, Johnsen S, Rasheed S, Makimura H, Lee H, et al. TNF-alpha antagonism with etanercept decreases glucose and increases the proportion of high molecular weight adiponectin in obese subjects with features of the metabolic syndrome. J Clin Endocrinol Metab. 2011;96(1):E146–50.
83. Yazdani-Biuki B, Mueller T, Brezinscheck HP, Hermann J, Graninger W, Wascher TC. Relapse of diabetes after interruption of chronic administration of anti-tumor necrosis factor-alpha antibody infliximab: a case observation. Diabetes Care. 2006;29(7):1712–3.
84. Kiortsis D, Mavridis A, Vasakos S, Nikas S, Drosos A. Effects of infliximab treatment on insulin resistance in patients with rheumatoid arthritis and ankylosing spondylitis. Ann Rheum Dis. 2005;64(5):765–6.
85. Yazdani-Biuki B, Stelzl H, Brezinscheck HP, Hermann J, Mueller T, Krippl P, et al. Improvement of insulin sensitivity in insulin resistant subjects during prolonged treatment with the anti-TNF-alpha antibody infliximab. Eur J Clin Invest. 2004;34(9):641–2.
86. Sloan-Lancaster J, Abu-Raddad E, Polzer J, Miller JW, Scherer JC, De Gaetano A, et al. Double-blind, randomized study evaluating the glycemic and anti-inflammatory effects of subcutaneous LY2189102, a neutralizing IL-1β antibody, in patients with type 2 diabetes. Diabetes Care. 2013;36(8):2239–46.
87. Cavelti-Weder C, Babians-Brunner A, Keller C, Stahel MA, Kurz-Levin M, Zayed H, et al. Effects of gevokizumab on glycemia and inflammatory markers in type 2 diabetes. Diabetes Care. 2012;35(8):1654–62.
88. Rissanen A, Howard CP, Botha J, Thuren T. Effect of anti-IL-1β antibody (canakinumab) on insulin secretion rates in impaired glucose tolerance or type 2 diabetes: results of a randomized, placebo-controlled trial. Diabetes Obes Metab. 2012;14(12):1088–96.

89. Ridker PM, Howard CP, Walter V, Everett B, Libby P, Hensen J, et al. Effects of interleukin-1β inhibition with canakinumab on haemoglobin A1c, lipids, C-reactive protein, interleukin-6, and fibrinogen: a phase IIb randomized, placebo-controlled trial. Circulation. 2012;126(23):2739–48.
90. van Asseldonk EJ, Stienstra R, Koenen TB, Joosten LA, Netea MG, Tack CJ. Treatment with Anakinra improves disposition index but not insulin sensitivity in nondiabetic subjects with the metabolic syndrome: a randomized, double-blind, placebo-controlled study. J Clin Endocrinol Metab. 2011;96(7):2119–26.
91. Goldfine AB, Conlin PR, Halperin F, Koska J, Permana P, Schwenke D, et al. A randomised trial of salsalate for insulin resistance and cardiovascular risk factors in persons with abnormal glucose tolerance. Diabetologia. 2013;56(4):714–23.
92. Goldfine AB, Fonseca V, Jablonski KA, Pyle L, Staten MA, Shoelson SE. The effects of salsalate on glycemic control in patients with type 2 diabetes: a randomized trial. Ann Intern Med. 2010;152(6):346–57.
93. Goldfine AB, Silver R, Aldhahi W, Cai D, Tatro E, Lee J, et al. Use of salsalate to target inflammation in the treatment of insulin resistance and type 2 diabetes. Clin Transl Sci. 2008;1(1):36–43.
94. Fleischman A, Shoelson SE, Bernier R, Goldfine AB. Salsalate improves glycemia and inflammatory parameters in obese young adults. Diabetes Care. 2008;31(2):289–94.
95. Ota K, Wildmann J, Ota T, Besedovsky HO, Del Rey A. Interleukin-1beta and insulin elicit different neuroendocrine responses to hypoglycemia. Ann N Y Acad Sci. 2009;1153:82–8.
96. Takasawa W, Ohnuma K, Hatano R, Endo Y, Dang NH, Morimoto C. Inhibition of dipeptidyl peptidase 4 regulates microvascular endothelial growth induced by inflammatory cytokines. Biochem Biophys Res Commun. 2010;401(1):7–12.
97. Donath MY. Targeting inflammation in the treatment of type 2 diabetes. Diabetes Obes Metab. 2013;15 Suppl 3:193–6.
98. Das A, Stroud S, Mehta A, Rangasamy S. New treatments for diabetic retinopathy. Diabetes Obes Metab. 2015;17(3):219–30.
99. Brown DM, Nguyen QD, Marcus DM, Boyer DS, Patel S, Feiner L, et al. Long-term outcomes of ranibizumab therapy for diabetic macular edema: the 36-month results from two phase III trials: RISE and RIDE. Ophthalmology. 2013;120(10):2013–22.
100. Diabetic Retinopathy Clinical Research Network. Randomized trial evaluating ranibizumab plus prompt or deferred laser or triamcinolone plus prompt laser for diabetic macular edema. Ophthalmology. 2010;117(6):1064–77.
101. Michaelides M, Kaines A, Hamilton RD, Fraser-Bell S, Rajendram R, Quhill F, et al. A prospective randomized trial of intravitreal bevacizumab or laser therapy in the management of diabetic macular edema (BOLT study) 12-month data: report 2. Ophthalmology. 2010;117(6):1078–86.

Chapter 4
Ischemic Stroke

Ana Catarina Fonseca, Diana Aguiar de Sousa, and José M. Ferro

Abstract In recent years, there was a surge in interest for biomarkers in ischemic stroke, with several purposes. In this chapter we will focus on biomarkers with potential use in ischemic stroke, namely, in diagnosis, grading of severity, identification of subtypes, and prediction of outcome or recurrence. A special emphasis will be placed on the role of inflammation in stroke, as it plays a key role in the cascade of events leading to progression of ischemic brain injury. However, the role of biomarkers in the clinical management of ischemic stroke is still limited. Therapeutic trials attempting to intervene on the inflammatory process are also briefly mentioned.

Keywords Ischemic stroke • Biomarkers • Inflammation • Diagnosis • Prognosis • Severity • S100B • Interleukins • MMP • CRP

A biomarker is defined as a molecular, biological, or physical characteristic that indicates a specific physiologic state. It is used in clinical practice to identify risk for disease, diagnose disease and its severity, guide intervention strategies, and monitor patient responses to therapy [1]. Biomarkers have been progressively recognized as important diagnostic tools. Ideally, a biomarker should be highly sensitive, specific, accessible, accurate, reproducible by an analytical method, cost-effective and have a result that can be easily interpreted by a physician.

In this chapter we will use the term biomarker in a restricted sense, as we will focus on molecular serum and CSF biomarkers, excluding genetic, clinical, and imaging biomarkers. We will perform a narrative review of the evidence supporting the use of blood and CSF biomarkers in the diagnosis of ischemic stroke; in grading the severity of stroke; in the identification of stroke subtypes, namely, cardioembolic strokes; and in predicting outcomes, including death, neurological deficit, functional outcomes, and recurrence. Special emphasis will be placed on inflamma-

A.C. Fonseca, M.D., Ph.D., M.P.H. • D.A. de Sousa, M.D., M.Sc.
Department of Neurology, Hospital de Santa Maria, University of Lisbon, Lisbon, Portugal

J.M. Ferro, M.D., Ph.D. (✉)
Department of Neurology, Hospital de Santa Maria, University of Lisbon,
Avenida Professor Egas Moniz, 1649-035 Lisbon, Portugal
e-mail: jmferro@fm.ul.pt

© Springer International Publishing Switzerland 2015

F. Palavra et al. (eds.), *Biomarkers of Cardiometabolic Risk, Inflammation and Disease*, DOI 10.1007/978-3-319-16018-4_4

tory biomarkers and on the role of inflammation in acute focal brain ischemia. Therapeutic trials attempting to intervene on inflammatory processes related to ischemic stroke are briefly mentioned.

Inflammation in Acute Ischemic Stroke

Inflammation plays a key role in the cascade of events that leads to the progression of ischemic brain injury. Ischemia and subsequent endothelial vessel, neuron, and glia necrosis lead to the initiation of several cellular and molecular events (Table 4.1). During acute ischemia several genes are upregulated, namely, genes for pro-inflammatory cytokines (interleukin [IL]-6, IL-8, tumor necrosis factor [TNF]-α), heat shock proteins, growth factors, and leukocyte adhesion molecules.

IL-1β and TNF-α are the cytokines that mediate the initial inflammatory response [2]. IL-1β and TNF-α subsequently induce a secondary inflammatory response, more lasting, mediated by IL-6 and IL-8. These cytokines play an important role in the development of acute-phase reactants, such as C-reactive protein (CRP) and fibrinogen, and in the release of cell adhesion molecules, which contribute to leukocyte aggregation and later adhesion to vascular wall [3]. The overexpression of IL-6

Table 4.1 Timing and pathophysiology of the main damaging events related with cerebral ischemia

Minutes	Energy failure	Excitotoxicity
	Increase in intracellular Ca^{2+}, Na^{+}, Cl^{-}	Peri-infarct depolarization
	Diffusion of glutamate and K^{+} in the extracellular space	Cell swelling
Hours	Generation of reactive oxygen species	Oxidative stress
	Increased inducible nitric oxide synthase (iNOS) activity	Nitrosative stress
	Free radicals damage membranes, mitochondria, and DNA	Early postischemic inflammation
	Free radicals activate caspases and inflammatory mediators	Early blood-brain barrier dysfunction
	Upregulation of adhesion molecules promotes leukocyte infiltration	Microvascular injury
	Microglial activation	
	Cytokine receptor activation	
	Upregulation of matrix proteases	
Days	Matrix protease activation	Late blood-brain barrier dysfunction
	Proapoptotic signaling and cytotoxic proteins	Late postischemic inflammation
		Apoptosis
		Remodeling

by microglia and astrocytes may have a dual role in acute ischemia, with potential neurotoxic and neuroprotective actions [4]. CRP and pentraxin 3 (PTX3) are members of the pentraxin family, which plays a major role in the human innate immune response. PTX3 activates the complement pathway and enhances macrophage and dendritic cell activity. Microglia is also activated after cerebral ischemia. Activated microglia secretes cytokines such as TNF-α and develops phagocytic and major histocompatibility complex (MCH) class II-restricted antigen presenting features. Microglia can also produce growth factors like brain-derived neurotrophic factor (BDNF) [5]. The inflammatory mediators that are produced during the innate immune response induce the expression of cellular adhesion molecules (CAMs) that mediate leukocyte recruitment, transendothelial migration, and adhesion to the vascular endothelium. Leukocytes present in the ischemic area produce more inflammatory mediators, which activate adaptive immune response [6].

All these inflammatory responses are an important determinant of the clinical outcome, lesion size, edema, and hemorrhagic transformation. The breakdown of the blood-brain barrier (BBB) allows the passage of some of these substances into the peripheral circulation and cerebrospinal fluid, where they can be measured. S100B is assumed to be a marker of generalized BBB dysfunction. S100B belongs to a multigene family of calcium-binding proteins. Peripherally found biomarkers related to inflammation may therefore be clinically useful in ischemic stroke.

Biomarkers in the Clinical Setting of Ischemic Stroke

Diagnosis of Acute Ischemic Stroke

About a third of patients who present with stroke-like symptoms have a stroke mimic. Although brain magnetic resonance imaging (MRI) with diffusion sequence may be very useful for stroke diagnosis, its sensitivity for ischemic stroke has been reported to be of 92 % with a specificity of 75 %. DWI-negative MRI was particularly associated with less severe stroke (NIHSS 4 vs. 7), posterior circulation location, higher prevalence of small vessel disease, and longer time from symptom onset to imaging (120 min vs. 109 min) [7]. Hence, biomarkers capable of identifying patients with ischemic stroke might be clinically useful.

One of the most promising biomarkers for acute ischemic stroke is S100B. S100B is a calcium-binding protein synthesized by astrocytes and expressed primarily by these cells in the central nervous system (CNS) and to a lesser extent by Schwann cells. In a normal status, the concentration of S100B is 40-fold higher in CSF than in serum. Serum S100B levels have been shown to be significantly increased following ischemic stroke from 10 h to 2–3 days after stroke onset [8]. Serum levels of S100B were pointed to be useful for distinguishing between posterior circulation strokes and nonvascular vertigo. Two observational prospective studies found statistically significant higher levels of S100B in patients with posterior circulation stroke than in patients with noncentral causes of vertigo [9, 10]. Receiver-operating characteristic analysis revealed a sensitivity of 94.4 % and a specificity of 31.8 % for detecting stroke in patients presenting with vertigo for S100B [9].

Higher plasma levels of TNF-α, IL-6, and IL-1β in acute ischemic stroke have been found mainly in cardioembolic strokes [11].

Cell adhesion molecules (CAMs) released into the bloodstream may also be useful for the diagnosis of ischemic stroke. Previous studies showed higher serum levels of soluble intercellular adhesion molecule-1 (sICAM-1) and soluble vascular cell adhesion molecule-1 (sVCAM-1) in stroke patients on admission, compared to healthy controls [12].

The diagnostic accuracy of a biomarker panel to diagnose acute stroke including MMP-9 and S100B was evaluated in a prospective multicenter trial – the Biomarker Rapid Assessment in Ischemic Injury (BRAIN) study [13]. Within a 3-year period, 1,146 patients presenting with symptoms suspicious for stroke were enrolled. The multivariate model was capable of only moderately differentiating between stroke patients and mimics. Setting a threshold to the 25th percentile, it was possible to show a sensitivity of 86 % and a specificity of 37 % for discriminating stroke patients from mimics [13].

Stroke Severity

The need for biomarkers (a "brain troponin") that can reflect the severity of real-time brain injury has increased with the development of acute stroke therapies. Such biomarker can speed up decisions regarding the appropriateness of chemical or mechanical revascularization.

Several biomarkers showed an association with stroke severity as indicated by a more severe clinical picture and a larger infarct volume. S100B has a positive correlation with total infarct volume [14] and admission National Institute of Health Stroke Scale (NIHSS) scores [15]. Increased S100B in blood is not specific for cerebral infarction, as increases occur in other neurologic diseases, like traumatic brain injury. Higher levels of glial fibrillary acidic protein (GFAP) [16] and IL-6 [17] are also associated with larger infarct volumes.

MMPs are implicated in numerous pathogenic mechanisms in acute ischemic stroke, including BBB disruption. MMP-9 serum level was significantly increased after stroke onset, correlating with infarct volume and stroke severity [18]. In acute ischemic stroke higher baseline blood MMP-9 levels are associated with thrombolysis failure [19].

In a recent study, adiponectin values at day 0 were positively associated with neurological severity as evaluated by the NIHSS at admission [20]. Neuron-specific enolase (NSE) was also significantly correlated with the degree of neurological deficit (NIHSS on admission) [21]. The expression of vascular endothelial growth factor (VEGF) was correlated with infarct volume and clinical disability (Scandinavian Stroke Scale) [22]. D-dimer levels at admission were also associated with total infarct volume in patients with acute ischemic stroke and atrial fibrillation

[23]. The excitatory neurotransmitter glutamate was associated with infarct growth [24]. Elevated neuropeptide proenkephalin A (PENK-A) concentrations were also associated with the severity of ischemic stroke, assessed by the NIHSS and modified Rankin Scale [25].

Hemorrhagic Transformation

Hemorrhagic transformation (HT) is more likely to occur with increasing infarct size, early recanalization, cardioembolic etiology, and use of recombinant tissue plasminogen activator (rtPA). Early HT (less than 24 h after stroke onset) has been associated to MMP-9 and MMP-2 activation. MMP-9 is a proteolytic enzyme involved in tissue remodeling [26]. These metalloproteinases damage the neurovascular unit and lead to BBB disruption. Delayed HT (more than 24 h after stroke onset) has been related to the activation of MMP-2, MMP-3, MMP-9, and endogenous tissue plasminogen activator, neuroinflammation, and factors that promote vascular remodeling [26].

Increased MMP-9 levels measured in plasma samples of patients before rtPA administration (>140 ng/ml) were associated with HT [27]. The sensitivity, specificity, and positive and negative predictive values for HT by MMP-9 levels > 140 ng/mL were 92 %, 74 %, 26 %, and 99 %, respectively. When plasma levels of cellular fibronectin (c-Fn) ≥ 3.6 μg/mL were used in combination with MMP-9 activity, the specificity increased to 87 % and the positive predictive value increased to 41 % [28]. c-Fn is a component of the basal lamina that is synthesized and secreted by endothelial cells. When the basal lamina is disrupted, c-Fn is released into the plasma, leading to the recruitment of leukocytes.

Vascular adhesion protein-1 (VAP-1), a cell surface and circulating enzyme involved in the recruitment of lymphocytes and neutrophils through its semicarbazide-sensitive amine oxidase (SSAO) activity, has also been shown to predict HT. In an observational, prospective study of 141 ischemic stroke patients, significantly higher levels of plasma VAP-1/SSAO activity were present in patients who subsequently experienced HT [29].

Malignant Middle Cerebral Artery Infarction

Space-occupying brain edema is a life-threatening complication in patients with large hemispheric stroke. In 80 % of patients it leads to death, and patients who survive have severe neurological deficits.

In a study of 51 patients admitted within 6 h after stroke symptom onset caused by proximal middle cerebral artery (MCA) occlusion, 16 developed a malignant MCA infarct. In these patients, a 12-h S100B value > 0.35 μg/L predicted malignant infarction with a sensitivity of 75 % and a specificity of 80 %. A 24-h value > 1.03 μg/L provided a sensitivity of 94 % and a specificity of 83 % [30].

In an observational, prospective study of 40 consecutive patients with malignant MCA infarctions and 35 controls with massive MCA infarctions, less than 70 years of age and matched by stroke severity on admission, plasma c-Fn levels greater than 16.6 μg/mL were associated with the development of malignant infarctions with a sensitivity of 90 %, specificity of 100 %, and negative and positive predictive values of 89 and 100 %, respectively [31].

There are discrepant results regarding the role of MMP-13 as an independent predictor of infarct growth 24 h after stroke onset. Although an association was initially shown, subsequent studies could not detect significant differences in MMP-13 blood levels after stroke compared with controls [32, 33].

Ischemic Stroke Recurrence

Elevated blood CRP levels are a predictor of the risk of cardiovascular events, as they are known to be associated to endothelial cell dysfunction and decreased production of nitric oxide [34]. In a nested case-control study derived from the Perindopril Protection Against Recurrent Stroke Study (PROGRESS), inflammatory markers associated with the acute-phase response (IL-6, TNF-α, CRP, and fibrinogen) were associated with risk of recurrent stroke (>3 years of outcome). However, these markers were dependent on each other in multivariate models, and once all were included, only TNF-α retained a borderline association [35]. In a study that included transient ischemic attack and minor stroke patients, CRP was not associated with recurrent vascular events [36]. Also, in the MITICO study, a multicentered prospective observational study designed to assess the prognostic value of markers of inflammation in relation to the risk of recurrence of ischemic stroke, CRP was not independently associated with recurrent ischemic stroke within the first year after the index event. Only baseline levels of IL-6>5 pg/mL and VCAM-1>1,350 ng/mL were associated with vascular disease recurrence risk (OR: 28.7; 95 % CI: 14.2–58.0 vs. OR: 4.1; 95 % CI: 2.4–7.1, respectively) following adjustment for confounding variables [37]. This independent association of IL-6 or VCAM-1 with stroke recurrence was not reproduced in further studies [38, 39].

The majority of studies that analyzed stroke recurrence combined different stroke etiologies. However, biomarker profiles regarding stroke recurrence may differ between lacunar stroke and other ischemic stroke subtypes. In the study Levels of Inflammatory Markers in the Treatment of Stroke (LIMITS), an international, multicenter, prospective biomarker study nested within Secondary Prevention of Small Subcortical Strokes (SPS3), a phase III trial in patients with recent lacunar stroke, among recent lacunar stroke patients, CRP levels predicted the risk of recurrent strokes. In patients with an initial lacunar stroke compared with the bottom quartile, those in the top quartile (CRP>4.86 mg/L) were at increased risk of recurrent ischemic stroke even after adjusting for demographics and risk factors (adjusted HR, 2.32; 95 % CI, 1.15–4.68) [40].

Lipoprotein-associated phospholipase A2 (Lp-PLA2) is an inflammatory biomarker that has been described as an independent risk marker for recurrent events in ischemic stroke [41]. Lp-PLA2 is an enzyme that hydrolyzes oxidized phospholipids, releasing lysophosphatidylcholine, that has pro-inflammatory properties. It is considered to be involved in the development of atherosclerosis and plaque rupture [41]. In 2005, the Lp-PLA2 blood test was approved by the US Food and Drug Administration (FDA) for assessing the risk of ischemic stroke [41].

The Northern Manhattan Stroke Study analyzed the predictive role of Lp-PLA2 drawn at the time of initial stroke in predicting the risk of recurrent stroke. In this population-based study of 467 patients with a first ischemic stroke, Lp-PLA2 conferred a 2.1-fold increase in recurrent stroke risk (HR, 2.08; 95 % CI, 1.04–4.18) [42].

Patients with elevated erythrocyte sedimentation rate (ESR) have been shown to have a greater risk of recurrence within 2 weeks of stroke onset [43].

Prognosis

Several studies have demonstrated an association between blood biomarkers of several pathophysiological processes and outcome after stroke. In most cases, however, it was not demonstrated if measurement of such biomarkers had an increment on prognostic accuracy over existing clinical and imaging predictors. This fact strongly limits their clinical significance [17].

Cardiac Biomarkers

A number of studies consistently found an increased mortality in stroke patients with increased cardiac troponin I or T [44–48], including the recent large biomarker substudy of the RE-LY trial (Randomized Evaluation of Long-Term Anticoagulation Therapy) [49]. Although some negative results were published [17], it was demonstrated in a retrospective study that adding troponin levels to a multivariate clinical model predicting long-term mortality increased the discriminative power of the model [50]. This effect persisted independently of traditional major coronary risk factors [51]. Some authors consider that troponin levels may reflect neurogenic cardiac damage, which is more frequent in severe strokes and is by itself a cause of acute stroke mortality. An ongoing prospective study in a large cohort of stroke patients is aiming to determine the causes of troponin elevation using coronary angiography [52, 53].

In a recent study with more than 400 patients, brain natriuretic peptide (BNP) was an independent prognostic marker for overall mortality in patients with ischemic stroke or TIA [54].

Inflammatory Biomarkers

In a recent meta-analysis evaluating the prognostic value of blood IL-6 in the prediction of functional outcome after stroke, standardized IL-6 levels in the 4th quartile were independently associated with a poor outcome (OR = 2.346). However, the additional predictive value of IL-6 was only moderate [55]. Higher levels of plasma IL-6 were also associated with death within the first 2 years after a stroke [56] and increased risk of future infection [56]. Higher MMP-9 levels were also correlated with functional outcomes [18].

CRP is an acute-phase-response protein, which may itself have pro-inflammatory effects and increase secondary brain injury. There is a significant association between elevated baseline high-sensitivity CRP levels and unfavorable long-term functional outcomes [57]. This association is present in a dose-related manner [58]. Elevated serum CRP levels in the acute and subacute phases (0–15 days) independently predicted mortality in several large cohort studies [58, 59], including in patients submitted to intravenous thrombolysis, regardless of vessel recanalization. However, measurement imprecision and confounding by infection and nonspecific inflammation are important limitations in considering CRP as a biomarker in acute stroke. The levels of fibrinogen that is also an acute-phase protein similarly are a predictor of poor functional outcome of stroke [60].

Elevated neuropeptide proenkephalin A (PENK-A) concentrations may have prognostic value for fatal and nonfatal events [25]. In one study, chemokines CCL17 and CCL22 showed a very faint power to discriminate patients who improve within the first 24–48 h after stroke from the remaining. Indeed, none of these chemokines seems to be a reliable prognostic biomarker in the hyperacute phase of stroke [61].

Other Biomarkers

Copeptin is a hypothalamic hormone derived from the precursor of vasopressin. Copeptin levels were shown to independently predict outcome and mortality in acute stroke. Also, in a multivariate model, copeptin improved significantly prediction when added to the NIHSS score and age [62]. The excitatory neurotransmitter glutamate is associated with poor outcome [24] and glial fibrillary acidic protein (GFAP) was positively correlated with the outcomes [16]. S100B blood levels at 48–96 h after stroke onset correlate positively with functional outcome in patients with nonlacunar MCA infarctions [63]. High plasma S100A12 levels on admission are associated with a poor outcome [64]. In a recent study, adiponectin values at day 0 were positively associated with poor outcome (modified Rankin Scale ≥ 3 on day 90) [20].

Trials of Immune Treatment in Acute Stroke

A few randomized controlled trials (RCT) have tested the hypothesis that intervening in the immune response within the ischemic cascade could improve stroke outcome. Unfortunately, despite all the encouraging results in basic science and animal models, results were deceiving as all these trials were negative. Enlimomab, a murine intercellular adhesion molecule 1 (ICAM-1) antibody, was tested against placebo in an RCT that included 625 patients treated within 6 h after stroke onset. Enlimomab was not effective and increased significantly the risk of infections and fever [65]. An adaptive dose-response trial of a neutrophil inhibitory factor succeeded to enroll 966 acute stroke patients, but was early terminated for futility [66]. An interleukin receptor antagonist was safe and well tolerated in acute stroke patients [67], but it was not tested in a phase III study. A trial of interferon beta completed enrollment, but results were not published [68, 69]. Arundic acid (ONO-2506), a novel modulator of astrocyte activation, was tested in a dose-escalating, randomized, double-blind phase I trial in 92 patients with acute ischemic stroke, within 24 h of stroke onset [70]. The study drug was infused for 1 h daily over 7 days. No dose-related pattern of serious adverse events was detected. In an exploratory efficacy analysis, a dose of 8 mg/kg/h produced a favorable trend in reduction of NIHSS score, needing confirmation in a future clinical trial, whose results were not published [71]. Minocycline is an antibiotic that acts via several pathways, including inhibition of microglial activation and reduction of T-cell migration. Minocycline was evaluated in a randomized controlled pilot trail including 95 patients treated within 24 h from stroke onset. The drug was safe, but not efficacious. A meta-analysis including this study and two other trials suggested that minocycline may increase the odds of survival free of handicap, but there was substantial heterogeneity between trials [72].

Conclusion

In recent years there was a surge in interest for biomarkers in ischemic stroke, with several purposes ranging from diagnosis to outcome prediction (Table 4.2). Despite all work done until now, the role of biomarkers in ischemic stroke management is very limited, and none can be recommended for routine use in clinical practice. Future research should focus not only on the identification of new biomarkers but also in the evaluation of panels of multiple biomarkers in large samples of ischemic stroke patients. Their value above existing demographic, clinical, and imaging variables and diagnostic tools should be proved.

Table 4.2 List of potential useful biomarkers for different ischemic stroke stages

Ischemic stroke	Potential biomarker
Diagnosis	S100B
	sICAM-1
	sVCAM-1
Severity	S100B
	NSE
	GFAP
	IL-6
	MMP-9
	Adiponectin
	VEGF
	D-dimer
	PENK-A
Hemorrhagic transformation	MMP-9
	c-Fn
	VAP-1/SSAO activity
Recurrence	CRP
	Lp-PLA2
	ESR
Malignant MCA infarction	S100B
	c-Fn
Prognosis	Copeptin
	IL-6
	MMP-9
	Troponin I or T
	Brain natriuretic peptide
	C-reactive protein
	Fibrinogen
	GFAP
	S100B
	S100A12
	Adiponectin

References

1. Altar CA. The Biomarkers Consortium: on the critical path of drug discovery. Clin Pharmacol Ther. 2008;83(2):361–4.
2. Smith CW. Endothelial adhesion molecules and their role in inflammation. Can J Physiol Pharmacol. 1993;71:76–87.
3. Rodríguez-Yáñez M, Castillo J. Role of inflammatory markers in brain ischemia. Curr Opin Neurol. 2008;21:353–7.
4. Muller B. Cytokine imbalance in non-immunological disease. Cytokine. 2002;18:334–9.
5. Doll DN, Barr TL, Simpkins JW. Cytokines: their role in stroke and potential use as biomarkers and therapeutic targets. Aging Dis. 2014;5:294–306.
6. Famakin BM. The immune response to acute focal cerebral ischemia and associated post-stroke immunodepression: a focused review. Aging Dis. 2014;5:307–26.

7. Simonsen CZ, Madsen MH, Schmitz ML, Mikkelsen IK, Fisher M, Andersen G. Sensitivity of diffusion- and perfusion-weighted imaging for diagnosing acute ischemic stroke is 97.5%. Stroke. 2015;46:98–101.
8. Nash DL, Bellolio MF, Stead LG. S100 as a marker of acute brain ischemia: a systematic review. Neurocrit Care. 2008;8:301–7.
9. Purrucker JC, Herrmann O, Lutsch JK, Zorn M, Schwaninger M, Bruckner T, et al. Serum protein S100β is a diagnostic biomarker for distinguishing posterior circulation stroke from vertigo of nonvascular causes. Eur Neurol. 2014;72:278–84.
10. Kartal AG, Yılmaz S, Yaka E, Pekdemir M, Sarisoy HT, Çekmen MB, et al. Diagnostic value of S100B protein in the differential diagnosis of acute vertigo in the emergency department. Acad Emerg Med. 2014;21:736–41.
11. Licata G, Tuttolomondo A, Di Raimondo D, Corrao S, Di Sciacca R, Pinto A. Immuno-inflammatory activation in acute cardio-embolic strokes in comparison with other subtypes of ischaemic stroke. Thromb Haemost. 2009;101:929–37.
12. Rallidis LS, Zolindaki MG, Vikelis M, Kaliva K, Papadopoulos C, Kremastinos DT. Elevated soluble intercellular adhesion molecule-1 levels are associated with poor short-term prognosis in middle-aged patients with acute ischaemic stroke. Int J Cardiol. 2009;132:216–20.
13. Laskowitz DT, Kasner SE, Saver J, Remmel KS, Jauch EC. Clinical usefulness of a biomarker-based diagnostic test for acute stroke: the Biomarker Rapid Assessment in Ischemic Injury (BRAIN) study. Stroke. 2009;40:77–85.
14. Missler U, Wiesmann M, Friedrich C, Kaps M. S-100 protein and neuron-specific enolase concentrations in blood as indicators of infarction volume and prognosis in acute ischemic. Stroke. 1997;28:1956–60.
15. Jauch EC, Lindsell C, Broderick J, Fagan SC, Tilley BC, Levine SR, NINDS rt-PA Stroke Study Group. Association of serial biochemical markers with acute ischemic stroke: the National Institute of Neurological Disorders and Stroke recombinant tissue plasminogen activator Stroke Study. Stroke. 2006;37:2508–13.
16. Herrmann M, Vos P, Wunderlich MT, de Bruijn CH, Lamers KJ. Release of glial tissue-specific proteins after acute stroke: a comparative analysis of serum concentrations of protein S-100B and glial fibrillary acidic protein. Stroke. 2000;31:2670–7.
17. Whiteley W, Wardlaw J, Dennis M, Lowe G, Rumley A, Sattar N, et al. The use of blood biomarkers to predict poor outcome after acute transient ischemic attack or ischemic stroke. Stroke. 2012;43:86–91.
18. Ramos-Fernandez M, Bellolio MF, Stead LG. Matrix metalloproteinase-9 as a marker for acute ischemic stroke: a systematic review. J Stroke Cerebrovasc Dis. 2011;20:47–54.
19. Heo JH, Kim SH, Lee KY, Kim EH, Chu CK, Nam JM. Increase in plasma matrix metalloproteinase-9 in acute stroke patients. Stroke. 2003;34:e48–50.
20. Kuwashiro T, Ago T, Kamouchi M, Matsuo R, Hata J, Kuroda J, et al. Significance of plasma adiponectin for diagnosis, neurological severity and functional outcome in ischemic stroke – Research for Biomarkers in Ischemic Stroke (REBIOS). Metabolism. 2014;63:1093–103.
21. Singh HV, Pandey A, Shrivastava AK, Raizada A, Singh SK, Singh N. Prognostic value of neuron specific enolase and IL-10 in ischemic stroke and its correlation with degree of neurological deficit. Clin Chim Acta. 2013;419:136–8.
22. Slevin M, Krupinski J, Slowik A, Kumar P, Szczudlik A, Gaffney J. Serial measurement of vascular endothelial growth factor and transforming growth factor-beta1 in serum of patients with acute ischemic stroke. Stroke. 2000;31:1863–70.
23. Matsumoto M, Sakaguchi M, Okazaki S, Furukado S, Tagaya M, Etani H, et al. Relationship between plasma (D)-dimer level and cerebral infarction volume in patients with nonvalvular atrial fibrillation. Cerebrovasc Dis. 2013;35:64–72.
24. Castellanos M, Sobrino T, Pedraza S, Moldes O, Pumar JM, Silva Y, et al. High plasma glutamate concentrations are associated with infarct growth in acute ischemic stroke. Neurology. 2008;71:1862–8.
25. Doehner W, von Haehling S, Suhr J, Ebner N, Schuster A, Nagel E, et al. Elevated plasma levels of neuropeptide proenkephalin a predict mortality and functional outcome in ischemic stroke. J Am Coll Cardiol. 2012;60:346–54.

26. Jickling GC, Liu D, Stamova B, Ander BP, Zhan X, Lu A, et al. Hemorrhagic transformation after ischemic stroke in animals and humans. J Cereb Blood Flow Metab. 2014;34:185–99.
27. Montaner J, Molina CA, Monasterio J, Abilleira S, Arenillas JF, Ribó M, et al. Matrix metalloproteinase-9 pretreatment level predicts intracranial hemorrhagic complications after thrombolysis in human stroke. Circulation. 2003;107:598–603.
28. Castellanos M, Sobrino T, Millan M, García M, Arenillas J, Nombela F, et al. Serum cellular fibronectin and matrix metalloproteinase-9 as screening biomarkers for the prediction of parenchymal hematoma after thrombolytic therapy in acute ischemic stroke: a multicenter confirmatory study. Stroke. 2007;38:1855–9.
29. Hernandez-Guillamon M, Garcia-Bonilla L, Solé M, Sosti V, Parés M, Campos M, et al. Plasma VAP-1/SSAO activity predicts intracranial hemorrhages and adverse neurological outcome after tissue plasminogen activator treatment in stroke. Stroke. 2010;41:1528–35.
30. Foerch C, Otto B, Singer OC, Neumann-Haefelin T, Yan B, Berkefeld J, et al. Serum S100B predicts a malignant course of infarction in patients with acute middle cerebral artery occlusion. Stroke. 2004;35:2160–4.
31. Serena J, Blanco M, Castellanos M, Silva Y, Vivancos J, Moro MA, et al. The prediction of malignant cerebral infarction by molecular brain barrier disruption markers. Stroke. 2005;36:1921–6.
32. Rosell A, Alvarez-Sabín J, Arenillas JF. A matrix metalloproteinase protein array reveals a strong relation between MMP-9 and MMP-13 with diffusion-weighted image lesion increase in human stroke. Stroke. 2005;36:1415–20.
33. Horstmann S, Kalb P, Koziol J, Gardner H, Wagner S. Profiles of matrix metalloproteinases, their inhibitors, and laminin in stroke patients: influence of different therapies. Stroke. 2003;34:2165–70.
34. Miao Y, Liao JK. Potential serum biomarkers in the pathophysiological processes of stroke. Expert Rev Neurother. 2014;14:173–85.
35. Welsh P, Lowe GD, Chalmers J, Campbell DJ, Rumley A, Neal BC, et al. Associations of proinflammatory cytokines with the risk of recurrent stroke. Stroke. 2008;39:2226–30.
36. Selvarajah JR, Smith CJ, Hulme S, Georgiou R, Sherrington C, Staniland J, et al. Does inflammation predispose to recurrent vascular events after recent transient ischaemic attack and minor stroke? The North West of England transient ischaemic attack and minor stroke (NORTHSTAR) study. Int J Stroke. 2011;6:187–94.
37. Castillo J, Alvarez-Sabin J, Martinez-Vila E, Montaner J, Sobrino T, Vivancos J, et al. Inflammation markers and prediction of poststroke vascular disease recurrence: the MITICO study. J Neurol. 2009;256:217–24.
38. Segal HC, Burgess AI, Poole DL, Mehta Z, Silver LE, Rothwell PM. Population-based study of blood biomarkers in prediction of subacute recurrent stroke. Stroke. 2014;45:2912–7.
39. Prugger C, Luc G, Haas B, Morange PE, Ferrieres J, Amouyel P, et al. PRIME Study Group. Multiple biomarkers for the prediction of ischemic stroke: the PRIME study. Arterioscler Thromb Vasc Biol. 2013;33:659–66.
40. Elkind MS, Luna JM, McClure LA, Zhang Y, Coffey CS, Roldan A, et al. C-reactive protein as a prognostic marker after lacunar stroke: levels of inflammatory markers in the treatment of stroke study. Stroke. 2014;45:707–16.
41. Gorelick PB. Lipoprotein-associated phospholipase A2 and risk of stroke. Am J Cardiol. 2008;101:34F–40.
42. Elkind MS, Tai W, Coates K, Paik MC, Sacco RL. High-sensitivity C-reactive protein, lipoprotein-associated phospholipase A2, and outcome after ischemic stroke. Arch Intern Med. 2006;166:2073–80.
43. Chamorro A, Vila N, Blanc R, Saiz A, Ascaso C, Deulofeu R. The prognostic value of acute phase response in stroke recurrence. Eur J Neurol. 1997;4:491–7.
44. Dixit S, Castle M, Velu RP, Swisher L, Hodge C, Jaffe AS. Cardiac involvement in patients with acute neurologic disease: confirmation with cardiac troponin I. Arch Intern Med. 2000;160:3153–8.

45. Christensen H, Johannesen HH, Christensen AF, Bendtzen K, Boysen G. Serum cardiac TnI in acute stroke is related to serum cortisol and TNF-alpha. Cerebrovasc Dis. 2004;18:194–9.
46. Di Angelantonio E, Fiorelli M, Toni D, Sacchetti ML, Lorenzano S, Falcou A, et al. Prognostic significance of admission levels of TnI in patients with acute ischaemic stroke. J Neurol Neurosurg Psychiatry. 2005;76:76–81.
47. James P, Ellis CJ, Whitlock RM, McNeil AR, Henley J, Anderson NE. Relation between troponin T concentration and mortality in patients presenting with an acute stroke: observational study. BMJ. 2000;320:1502–4.
48. Jensen JK, Kristensen SR, Bak S, Atar D, Hoilund-Carlsen PF, Mickley H. Frequency and significance of troponin T elevation in acute ischemic stroke. Am J Cardiol. 2007;99:108–12.
49. Hijazi Z, Oldgren J, Andersson U, Connolly SJ, Ezekowitz MD, Hohnloser SH, et al. Cardiac biomarkers are associated with an increased risk of stroke and death in patients with atrial fibrillation. A randomized evaluation of long-term anticoagulation therapy (RE-LY) substudy. Circulation. 2012;125:1605–16.
50. Faiz KW, Thommessen B, Einvik G, Omland T, Ronning OM. Prognostic value of high-sensitivity cardiac troponin T in acute ischemic stroke. J Stroke Cerebrovasc Dis. 2014;23:241–8.
51. Hijazi Z, Oldgren J, Siegbahn A, Granger CB, Wallentin L. Biomarkers in atrial fibrillation: a clinical review. Eur Heart J. 2013;34:1475–80.
52. Scheitz JF, Mochmann HC, Nolte CH, Haeusler KG, Audebert HJ, Heuschmann PU, et al. Troponin elevation in acute ischemic stroke (TRELAS) – protocol of a prospective observational trial. BMC Neurol. 2011;11:98.
53. Faiz KW, Thommessen B, Einvik G, Brekke PH, Omland T, Rønning OM. Determinants of high sensitivity cardiac troponin T elevation in acute ischemic stroke. BMC Neurol. 2014;14:96.
54. Nigro N, Wildi K, Mueller C, Schuetz P, Mueller B, Fluri F, et al. BNP but Not s-cTnln is associated with cardioembolic aetiology and predicts short and long term prognosis after cerebrovascular events. PLoS One. 2014;9:e102704.
55. Bustamante A, Sobrino T, Giralt D, García-Berrocoso T, Llombart V, Ugarriza I, et al. Prognostic value of blood interleukin-6 in the prediction of functional outcome after stroke: a systematic review and meta-analysis. J Neuroimmunol. 2014;274:215–24.
56. Kwan J, Horsfield G, Bryant T, Gawne-Cain M, Durward G, Byrne CD, et al. IL-6 is a predictive biomarker for stroke associated infection and future mortality in the elderly after an ischemic stroke. Exp Gerontol. 2013;48:960–5.
57. VanGilder RL, Davidov DM, Stinehart KR, Huber JD, Turner RC, Wilson KS, et al. C-reactive protein and long-term ischemic stroke prognosis. J Clin Neurosci. 2014;21:547–53.
58. Montaner J, Fernandez-Cadenas I, Molina CA, Ribó M, Huertas R, Rosell A, et al. Poststroke C-reactive protein is a powerful prognostic tool among candidates for thrombolysis. Stroke. 2006;37:1205–10.
59. Huang Y, Jing J, Zhao XQ, Wang CX, Wang YL, Liu GF, et al. High-sensitivity C-reactive protein is a strong risk factor for death after acute ischemic stroke among Chinese. CNS Neurosci Ther. 2012;18:261–6.
60. Hasan N, McColqan P, Edwards RJ, Sharma P. Towards the identification of blood biomarkers for acute stroke in humans: a comprehensive systematic review. Br J Clin Pharmacol. 2012;74:230–40.
61. García-Berrocoso T, Giralt D, Llombart V, Bustamante A, Penalba A, Flores A, et al. Chemokines after human ischemic stroke: from neurovascular unit to blood using protein arrays. Transl Proteomics. 2014;3:1–9.
62. De Marchis GM, Katan M, Weck A, Fluri F, Foerch C, Findling O, et al. Copeptin adds prognostic information after ischemic stroke: results from the CoRisk study. Neurology. 2013;80:1–9.
63. Foerch C, Singer OC, Neumann-Haefelin T, du Mesnil de Rochemont R, Steinmetz H, Sitzer M. Evaluation of serum S100B as a surrogate marker for long-term outcome and infarct volume in acute middle cerebral artery infarction. Arch Neurol. 2005;62:1130–4.

64. Wakisaka Y, Ago T, Kamouchi M, Kuroda J, Matsuo R, Hata J, et al. Plasma S100A12 is associated with functional outcome after ischemic stroke: research for Biomarkers in Ischemic Stroke. J Neurol Sci. 2014;340:75–9.
65. Enlimomab Acute Stroke Trial Investigators. Use of anti-ICAM-1 therapy in ischemic stroke: results of the Enlimomab Acute Stroke Trial. Neurology. 2001;57:1428–34.
66. Krams M, Lees KR, Hacke W, Grieve AP, Orgogozo JM, Ford GA. ASTIN Study Investigators. Acute Stroke Therapy by Inhibition of Neutrophils (ASTIN): an adaptive dose-response study of UK-279,276 in acute ischemic stroke. Stroke. 2003;34:2543–8.
67. Emsley HC, Smith CJ, Georgiou RF, Vail A, Hopkins S, Rothwell N, et al. A randomised phase II study of interleukin-1 receptor antagonist in acute stroke patients. J Neurol Neurosurg Psychiatry. 2005;76:1366–72.
68. Ferro JM, Dávalos A. Other neuroprotective therapies on trial in acute stroke. Cerebrovasc Dis. 2006;21 Suppl 2:127–30.
69. National Institute of Neurological Disorders and Stroke (NINDS). Recombinant human interferon beta-1a in acute ischemic stroke: a dose escalation and safety study. In: ClinicalTrials.gov [Internet]. Bethesda: National Library of Medicine (US); 2014. Available from: https://clinicaltrials.gov/ct2/show/NCT00097318.
70. Pettigrew LC, Kasner SE, Albers GW, Gorman M, Grotta JC, Sherman DG, Funakoshi Y, Ishibashi H, Arundic Acid (ONO-2506) Stroke Study Group. Safety and tolerability of arundic acid in acute ischemic stroke. J Neurol Sci. 2006;251:50–6.
71. Ono Pharma USA Inc. A study to evaluate the effects of ONO-2506 intravenous infusion in patients with acute ischemic stroke. In: ClinicalTrials.gov [Internet]. Bethesda: National Library of Medicine (US); 2014. Available from: https://clinicaltrials.gov/show/NCT00046761.
72. Kohler E, Prentice DA, Bates TR, Hankey GJ, Claxton A, van Heerden J, Blacker D. Intravenous minocycline in acute stroke: a randomized, controlled pilot study and meta-analysis. Stroke. 2013;44:2493–9.

Chapter 5
Chronic Kidney Disease

Alice Santos-Silva, Elísio Costa, and Rui Alves

Abstract The identification of reliable biomarkers of early kidney injury and of progression of the disease, as well as the identification of predictive biomarkers of morbidity and mortality, is an emergent area of research in the clinical area of nephrology. The more promising new biomarkers of kidney function, of the pathophysiological process underlying renal impairment, and of the associated cardiovascular risk are reviewed. Because inflammation is a common feature of kidney disease, inflammation as a risk factor and target for therapy in kidney disease will be also addressed and the inflammatory biomarkers reviewed.

Keywords Biomarkers • Kidney disease • Inflammation • Kidney function • Renal injury

Biomarkers of Kidney Disease

During the last few decades, there have been several advances in the management of chronic kidney disease (CKD) patients and in dialysis techniques; however, the mortality continues unacceptably high in CKD patients. The identification of reliable biomarkers of early kidney injury and of progression of the disease, as well as the identification of predictive biomarkers of morbidity and mortality, is, therefore, an emergent area of research in this clinical area.

Several newer biomarkers of CKD have been proposed more recently, to detect changes underlying the disease, namely, changes in kidney function, glomerular injury, tubulointerstitial injury, inflammation, fibrosis, and endothelial (dys)

A. Santos-Silva, Ph.D. (✉) • E. Costa, Ph.D.
UCIBIO, REQUIMTE, Laboratory of Biochemistry, Department of Biological Sciences, Faculty of Pharmacy, University of Porto, Rua Jorge Viterbo Ferreira, 228, Porto 4050-313, Portugal
e-mail: assilva@ff.up.pt

R. Alves, M.D., Ph.D.
Universitary Nephrology Unit, Faculty of Medicine, University of Coimbra, Coimbra, Portugal

© Springer International Publishing Switzerland 2015
F. Palavra et al. (eds.), *Biomarkers of Cardiometabolic Risk, Inflammation and Disease*, DOI 10.1007/978-3-319-16018-4_5

function [1]. These markers could be used for earlier diagnosis, for prognosis, to monitor the disease and to predict associated complications, as cardiovascular diseases. The biomarkers that are usually used in clinical practice for diagnosis and prognosis of CKD are markers of kidney function. Indeed, the traditional biomarkers of kidney function, estimated glomerular filtration rate, blood urea nitrogen, serum creatinine, albuminuria, and proteinuria, are the more commonly used. These widely used biomarkers of kidney function show increased values only after the biological changes underlying the functional renal impairment. Moreover, these biomarkers have no disease specificity. To overcome this, promising biomarkers, including more sensitive biomarkers of kidney function and more specific of the underlying pathophysiological process, have been proposed for CKD progression and for its associated complications. The newer biomarkers, by providing earlier diagnosis of kidney injury, would be very important, as a delay in the clinical diagnosis of kidney injury may severely affect the therapeutic approach to the patient.

Definition, Classification, and Prediction of Chronic Kidney Disease

CKD is a gradual and, usually, permanent loss of kidney function, over months to years, that can result from primary diseases of the kidneys. However, the major causes of kidney injury are secondary to other diseases, as diabetes, high blood pressure, inflammation, postinfectious conditions, systemic lupus erythematosus, use of analgesics over long time periods, human immunodeficiency virus infection, sickle cell disease, heroin abuse, amyloidosis, chronic kidney infections, polycystic kidney disease, and some cancers [2]. In the earlier stages of kidney disease, as the patients are often asymptomatic, the disease is, usually, detected during the evaluation of comorbid conditions and may be reversible in case of precocious diagnosis and treatment. In the later stages of CKD, the symptoms reflect the complications of decreased kidney function and, when severe, can only be treated by dialysis or transplantation. The identification of patients at earlier stages of CKD, followed by an appropriate management by specialized kidney services, should, therefore, lead to important clinical benefits.

According to the recent "Kidney Disease: Improving Global Outcomes" (KDIGO) Guidelines [3], CKD is defined as abnormalities of kidney structure or function, present for more than 3 months, with implications for health (Table 5.1), and is classified based on the cause of the disease, the estimated glomerular filtration rate (eGFR) class, and albuminuria (Table 5.2). This classification enables the clinicians to identify the risk for adverse outcomes, as worsening of renal dysfunction or even death. Actually, it is recommended to identify factors associated with CKD progression, namely, the cause of CKD, the levels of eGFR and albuminuria, age, sex, race/ethnicity, elevated blood pressure, hyperglycemia, dyslipidemia, smoking, obesity, history of cardiovascular disease (CVD), ongoing exposure to nephrotoxic agents, and others that could be useful for prognosis. As some of these

Table 5.1 Criteria for CKD

Markers of kidney damage (one or more)
Albuminuria
Urine sediment abnormalities
Electrolyte and other abnormalities due to tubular disorders
Abnormalities detected by histology
Structural abnormalities detected by imaging
History of kidney transplantation
Decreased GFR (GFR categories G3a–G5)

Adapted from KDIGO 2012 [3]

Abbreviations: *CKD* chronic kidney disease, *GFR* glomerular filtration rate

Table 5.2 Likelihood of chronic kidney disease, based on cause, glomerular filtration rate, and albuminuria

Cause	Category	eGFR	Albuminuria (proteinuria)		
Glomerular disease	1	≥90	A1 (<30)	A2 (30–300)	A3 (>300)
Tubulointerstitial disease	2	60–89	–	+	++
Vascular disease	3a	45–59	+	++	+++
	3b	30–45	++	+++	+++
Congenital disease	4	15–29	+++	+++	+++
Cystic disease	5	<15	+++	+++	+++

Adapted from KDIGO 2012 [3]

risk factors are modifiable, they should be identified and treated, as they may have impact on long-term outcomes, namely, in cardiovascular condition, quality of life, and progression of CKD [3].

Both albuminuria and eGFR are useful markers of CKD progression and are synergistic; thus, they should be used to monitor the disease, especially in patients with lower eGFR and higher albumin values (1–3 months), as they are more prone to worsening of the disease; they should be also used when clinical events occur that might have impact in renal function. The frequency of these measurements should be individualized, based on the patient's history and underlying cause of kidney disease. The regular monitoring of stable patients may include more frequent monitoring than annually, according to the underlying cause, history, eGFR, and albumin/creatinine ratio previously estimated.

Newer Biomarkers of Chronic Kidney Disease

The early identification of individuals at risk for CKD progression is very important, as it may delay or avoid its progression to end-stage kidney disease (ESKD). Besides albuminuria and eGFR, there are several biomarkers that have been included in clinical studies to evaluate its potential as markers for CKD progression.

The CaNPREDDICT, a Canadian study for prediction of risk and evaluation to dialysis, death, and interim cardiovascular events over time, is testing biomarkers 6 monthly in 2,500 prevalent patients with eGFR 15–45 ml/min in 50 centers across Canada over 36 months. After 1 year of follow-up, this group has recently reported [4] that most of the newer biomarkers did not improve the prediction of renal replacement therapy, when added to conventional risk factors such as eGFR, urine albumin to creatinine ratio, hemoglobin, phosphate, and albumin; however, N-terminal of the prohormone brain natriuretic peptide (NT-proBNP), fibroblast growth factor (FGF23), high-sensitivity (hs) CRP, and cystatin C significantly improved the prediction of death within 1 year.

The Spanish NEFRONA project is a prospective observational study involving 2,661 patients that aims to study the usefulness of imaging techniques and novel biomarkers in the prediction of cardiovascular risk in patients with CKD [5]. Other studies including the MMKD (Mild to Moderate Kidney Disease) [6], the CRIC (Chronic Renal Insufficiency Cohort), and the CRIB (Chronic Renal Impairment in Birmingham) evaluated a wide range of traditional and nontraditional cardiovascular risk biomarkers in CKD [7].

From these and other studies, several promising biomarkers have been proposed for CKD progression and for its associated comorbidities and mortality. These markers may also provide valuable data about the underlying pathophysiology of the disease [1], as they may be biomarkers of kidney function, glomerular injury, or tubulointerstitial injury.

Biomarkers of Kidney Function

Several molecules involved in kidney function, signaling, and structure have been evaluated as potential markers for CKD. The biomarkers currently used in clinical practice for the diagnosis and prognosis of CKD are markers of loss of kidney function. The most widely used are the eGFR, serum creatinine, blood urea nitrogen, and albuminuria or proteinuria. These markers indicate impaired renal function but have no disease specificity, and detectable changes in their concentration only appear after the biological changes in the organ causing the functional impairment.

The most important new biomarkers for kidney function include cystatin C [8], a small protein filtered and metabolized after tubular absorption, and the beta-trace protein [9], a lipocalin glycoprotein, which is a sensitive marker of glomerular filtration. According to the MMKD study, both are good markers of CKD progression; however, cystatin C seems to be more sensitive. Uric acid has also emerged as a novel and potentially modifiable risk factor for the development and progression of CKD; however, it is not currently clear whether hyperuricemia plays a causative role in CKD progression or is merely a biomarker of reduced kidney function [10].

Biomarkers of Tubulointerstitial Injury

Markers of renal tubular injury are not used routinely to describe kidney function and little is known about the risk of cardiovascular events and death associated with these biomarkers. Neutrophil gelatinase-associated lipocalin (NGAL), kidney injury molecule 1 (KIM-1), N-acetyl-β-D-glucosaminidase (NAG), liver-type fatty acid-binding protein (L-FABP), tenascin, and the tissue inhibitor of metalloproteinase 1 (TIMP-1) have emerged as potential biomarkers of tubulointerstitial injury.

According to the CRIC study [11], involving 3,386 participants, urine levels of NGAL were associated independently with future ischemic atherosclerotic events, but not with heart failure events or deaths. The Multi-Ethnic Study of Atherosclerosis (MESA), involving 686 participants, evaluated both NGAL and KIM-1 as markers of tubular injury and found that urinary KIM-1 level was associated with future risk of kidney disease independent of albuminuria and that both biomarkers are a promising tool for identifying persons at risk of CKD [12].

KIM-1 is a transmembrane tubular protein that is not found in healthy people, emerging therefore as a potential biomarker of kidney disease. It has been reported that KIM-1 is upregulated in patients with renal cell carcinoma, urate nephropathy, acute and chronic tubular injury, allograft nephropathy, and acute kidney injury after cardiac surgery. Actually, KIM-1 has been also reported as an independent predictor of graft loss in renal transplant recipients [13] and as a good marker to monitor potentially nephrotoxic therapies.

NAG is a lysosomal enzyme that is present in proximal tubular cells and is widely used to evaluate tubular renal function. NAG has a high molecular weight, which does not permit its filtration through the glomerular basal membrane and is rapidly cleared from the circulation by the liver. Thus, urinary NAG originates primarily from the proximal tubule, and increased urinary excretion is a consequence of renal tubular cell breakdown; its urinary excretion is, therefore, almost constant with minimal diurnal changes. The urinary NAG values should be expressed as a ratio to urinary creatinine concentration, as this relationship shows less variability than the urinary enzyme excretions related to volume or time.

NGAL is another biomarker of renal tubular injury that belongs to the superfamily of lipocalins, a group of iron-carrying proteins [13]. It was firstly reported to be produced by neutrophils, but it is also expressed in other tissues, such as kidney, liver, epithelial cells, and vascular cells in atherosclerotic plaques [14]. When tubular injury occurs, the expression of NGAL rises and is rapidly secreted; urine and plasma concentrations increase proportionally to severity and duration of renal injury and its concentration rapidly decreases with attenuation of renal injury.

There are different commercially available ELISA kits to evaluate NGAL. As it was found that NGAL is ultrafiltered and absorbed by polysulfone membranes, the NGAL blood levels may be reduced in patients under therapeutic hemodialysis using such type of membranes for the hemodialysis procedure; a moderate to severe inflammatory condition, coexisting with kidney injury, may be also a confounding factor in NGAL measurement, as the activation of neutrophils will contribute to increase the NGAL blood levels.

Several clinical studies and systematic reviews proposed NGAL as a reliable diagnostic and prognostic biomarker for kidney injury. A multicenter analysis of pooled data [15], including 2,322 critically ill children and adults, evaluated the prognostic value of acute kidney injury detected by NGAL and found that about 20 % of the patients presented an early increase in the concentration of NGAL, in the absence of diagnostic increases in serum creatinine. The increase in NGAL levels, usually, occurs 24–72 h before the increase in creatinine to diagnosis values. Thus, NGAL evaluation seems to be a useful early biomarker of kidney injury. Moreover, this study group showed that NGAL is also a useful prognostic biomarker, as patients with increased NGAL were at greater risk of adverse outcomes, including death, renal replacement therapy, and hospitalization, both in the presence and absence of an increase in serum creatinine levels. However, future prospective studies are needed to confirm histopathological agreement of NGAL with tubular injury, already shown in animal models; further studies are also needed to test whether NGAL-based early diagnosis of kidney injury leads to more successful and prompt therapeutic intervention and to improve the outcome of the patients. Indeed, in the absence of an early detection of kidney injury, the therapeutic intervention could only be delivered late in the course of AKI, with worsening of the disease and of its outcome.

L-FABP is a newly emerging biomarker that has antioxidant properties and is expressed in the cytoplasm of human renal proximal tubules. Its expression is upregulated and its urinary excretion is increased by various stressors, including urinary protein, hyperglycemia, tubular ischemia, toxins, and salt-sensitive hypertension, which lead to the progression of kidney disease [16]. Urinary L-FABP levels accurately reflect the degree of tubulointerstitial damage and are strongly correlated with the prognosis of CKD patients [17]. Concerning AKI, urinary L-FABP seems to be able to detect kidney injury before an increase in serum creatinine occurs. Urinary L-FABP may be also useful for the early detection of diabetic nephropathy, the leading cause of CKD. In a longitudinal study, a higher level of urinary L-FABP was found to be a risk factor for the progression of diabetic nephropathy. A recent single-center, prospective observational study reported that urinary L-FABP may be also a useful predictor of adverse long-term outcomes in kidney transplant patients [18].

Tenascin and TIMP-1 have also been proposed as biomarkers of tubulointerstitial injury; however, there are still few studies supporting their value. Tenascin has emerged as an important extracellular matrix, playing an important role in nephrogenesis and in several pathological processes in glomerulus and tubulointerstitial renal cells. TIMP-1 is a physiological inhibitor of matrix-degrading enzymes, namely, collagenase, gelatinase, and stromelysin. Patients with CKD present elevated serum and urinary levels of both tenascin and TIMP-1; however, the urinary levels did not correlate with the degree of proteinuria [19].

These biomarkers of tubulointerstitial injury may be used as earlier markers of AKI, as markers of the underlying predominant kidney injury in CKD, as well as markers of progression and outcome.

Biomarkers of Glomerular Injury

Proteinuria is widely used as a marker of glomerular function. More recently, new biomarkers of kidney podocyte injury, including urinary nephrin, podocin, and podocalyxin, have emerged as biomarkers of glomerular injury.

Podocytes are differentiated epithelial cells covering the outer surface of the glomerular capillaries, presenting interdigitating foot processes and forming narrow slits to provide a pathway for glomerular filtration. They act as a size and charge barrier to anionic proteins, due to the presence of podocalyxin, a negatively charged apical membrane protein. The injury of podocytes may lead to a reduced foot process and proteinuria, while the detachment of podocytes from the glomerular basement membrane leads to progression of glomerular diseases. Podocyte injury might be induced by angiotensin II, hyperglycemia, oxidative stress, infections, deposition of antigen-antibody complexes, mechanical stretch, and drugs. In these conditions, urinary levels of nephrin, podocin, and podocalyxin are increased and, therefore, may be used in a noninvasive way, as useful markers of glomerular function. Moreover, the evaluation of the number of urinary podocytes can provide real-time data about the number of podocytes detached in a certain period of time; thus, urinary podocyte count may be also used as a marker of ongoing glomerular injuries. According to Hanamura et al. [20] a decrease in the number of glomerular podocytes is associated with glomerulosclerosis, decline in renal function, and impaired selectivity of proteinuria, suggesting a causative relationship between detachment and loss of podocytes and progression of renal dysfunction. Urinary podocyte excretion was associated with proteinuria and active histological lesions. These biomarkers are promising and more specific of glomerular injury; however, further studies are needed to assess their values in clinical practice.

Biomarkers of Endothelial Dysfunction

Asymmetric dimethylarginine (ADMA) is a naturally occurring amino acid found in tissues and cells, acting as an endogenous inhibitor of the nitric oxide synthase, impairing the ability of nitric oxide for vasodilation, and is excreted in urine. Several studies have suggested that plasma concentration of ADMA provides a marker of risk for endothelial dysfunction and cardiovascular disease. ADMA blood levels are increased in patients with CKD (stages 1–5 with or without proteinuria) [21] and seem to provide a biomarker for CKD progression [22]; furthermore, it has been associated with CVD complications [23]. Thus, ADMA concentration has been proposed as a biomarker for endothelial dysfunction and for increased risk of cardiovascular mortality and morbidity, as well as a prognostic marker for the loss of renal function.

A recent prospective controlled 1-year follow-up study [24] on the effects of ADMA and other variables related to ADMA metabolism on the progression of kidney dysfunction, in 181 patients with CKD stages 3–5, showed that elevated ADMA was a strong predictor of progression only for patients with eGFR between 25 and 40 mL/min/1.73 m^2 (the borderline of CKD stages 3–4).

To evaluate ADMA blood levels, enzyme-linked immunosorbent assays have been mostly used; however, a recent study showed that these measurements overestimated ADMA levels in eGFR < 30 mL/min, as compared to the gold-standard liquid chromatography-electrospray tandem mass spectrometry.

Inflammation in Chronic Kidney Disease

A persistent low-grade inflammation is a common feature in CKD patients [25], which is usually enhanced in ESKD patients and even more enhanced in case of resistance to therapy with erythropoietic stimulating agents [26]. Emerging evidence also suggests that low-grade persistent inflammation magnifies other common features of the uremic phenotype, such as atherosclerosis, depression, protein-energy wasting, and vascular calcification, acting as a catalyst of the vicious circle of risk factors for ESKD.

The increased urinary proteins *per se* seem to induce proinflammatory and profibrotic changes, leading to tubulointerstitial damage through several pathways, namely, by inducing tubular cytokine expression and complement activation, which will induce infiltration of inflammatory cells in the interstitium and fibrinogenesis [25].

Inflammation is a major driving force of the uremic phenotype and circulating inflammatory biomarkers seem to be sensitive predictors for the outcome of CKD patients. Actually, several studies have demonstrated an association between biomarkers of systemic inflammation, namely, C-reactive protein (CRP), interleukin-6 (IL-6), tumor necrosis factor-α (TNF-α) [27–29], and fibrinogen [30], with lower kidney function. Moreover, several inflammatory markers have been shown to be associated with a higher risk for cardiovascular events and for mortality [31, 32]. CKD is accepted as an independent risk factor for CVD. Actually, most of the mild to moderate CKD patients die from CVD events, even before they need kidney replacement treatment [33].

The Framingham Offspring cohort study [34] involving 3,294 patients who attended the seventh examination cycle (1998–2001) evaluated several inflammatory markers, such as CRP, TNF-α, IL-6, TNF-α receptor 2 (TNFR2), intercellular adhesion molecule-1 (ICAM-1), monocyte chemoattractant protein-1 (MCP-1), P-selectin, CD-40 ligand, osteoprotegerin, urinary isoprostanes, myeloperoxidase, and fibrinogen, and showed that TNF-α, IL-6, TNFR2, MCP-1, osteoprotegerin, myeloperoxidase, and fibrinogen were higher in CKD patients.

The role of persistent inflammation as a potential cause for this high mortality rate triggered an increasing interest in inflammatory biomarkers for diagnosis, prognosis, and monitoring of CKD, as well as possible therapeutic targets.

C-Reactive Protein

CRP is a member of the family of pentraxins, which are small pentameric innate immunity effector proteins that are absent or weakly expressed in healthy conditions. Its synthesis by hepatocytes is induced by proinflammatory cytokines, such as IL-1, IL-6, and TNF-α. The plasmatic levels of CRP are widely used by clinicians to assess infectious or noninfectious types of systemic inflammation, and nephrologists recognize CRP levels as a useful biomarker for the outcome of CKD and ESKD patients. Several studies, such as the Jackson Heart study and the CARE (Cholesterol and Recurrent Events) trial, showed that plasma concentrations of CRP were associated with the presence of CKD and with a higher rate of kidney function decline, respectively [1].

CRP values show time-dependent variability, as they might be influenced by intercurrent clinical events, including comorbidities, infections, and changes in blood volume. Therefore, the motorization of CRP value is especially important when using CRP as a biomarker for the evolution of the disease and for the outcome of the patient. The persistence of high CRP values (from 3 to 6 months) marks a worst survival in CKD and in ESKD patients.

The prevalence of the utilization of CRP measurement varies across countries and dialysis facilities; however, according to the Dialysis Outcomes and Practice Patterns Study (DOPPS) III, there has been an increasing use of CRP measurement in nearly all countries [35]. This study hypothesized that the evaluation of CRP as a marker of underlying infection/inflammation in dialysis facilities could lead to lower adverse outcomes for the dialyzed patients. It was found that the measurement of CRP in the majority of patients within a dialysis facility (vs. less than 50 % of patients) was significantly related to a lower cardiovascular mortality, for facilities measuring CRP in at least 50 % of its patients. This finding strongly suggests that a more prevalent measurement of CRP may influence patient outcomes. Indeed, the use of a CRP screening for inflammation would trigger the evaluation of the possible underlying causes, when a rise in CRP value occurs, allowing a rapid clinical intervention and, therefore, an effective improvement in patient outcome. Moreover, this study confirmed that higher CRP values are associated with all-cause mortality and showed that this relationship with mortality was independent of the correlation with other common inflammatory markers.

Interleukin-6

Of all the acute-phase proteins and plasma biomarkers of inflammation, CRP is the most widely used. CRP is rapidly synthesized in hepatocytes, following an inflammatory stimulus by IL-6 during the acute phase of inflammation. Il-6 is a proinflammatory cytokine released by a variety of activated cell types, which has multiple cell targets and regulates the hepatic acute-phase response, promoting the synthesis of positive acute-phase reactants and inhibiting that of negative acute-phase reactants. IL-6 also controls several homeostatic functions including glucose metabolism, the hypothalamic-pituitary-adrenal axis, affecting mood, fatigue and depression, and hematopoiesis. A systemic increase in IL-6 causes hyperthermia and leads to a general loss of activity and appetite.

Several comparative studies showed that IL-6 might be better prognostic and stratification marker of CKD than other molecules, including CRP and TNF-α [36]. However, although sensitive, the evaluation of IL-6 is still not routinely used in clinical monitoring.

Soluble Tumor Necrosis Factor Receptor 2

TNF-α is a proinflammatory agonist mediator that is produced in a wide variety of innate and adaptive immune responses, including CKD. It binds to cell surface receptors on target cells and induces expression of adhesion molecules, chemokines for leukocytes, and apoptosis in susceptible cells. Soluble TNFR2 (sTNFR2) are increased in the setting of inflammation and of CKD. Thus, TNF-α appears to mediate progressive renal injury, and both sTNFR2 and CRP may be used as markers of inflammation. As referred, data from the CARE trial showed that plasma concentration of CRP and also sTNFR2 at baseline were independently associated with a higher kidney function decline [1].

Pentraxin 3

Pentraxin 3 (PTX3) is a long pentraxin that belongs to the same pentraxin superfamily of acute-phase reactants, as CRP. PTX3 is produced by both resident and innate immunity cells (vascular endothelial cells, smooth muscle cells, fibroblasts, adipocytes, macrophages, and dendritic cells) in the peripheral tissues, increasing rapidly in response to primary local activation of inflammation. Thus, in contrast to short pentraxins (such as CRP), which are only expressed by hepatocytes, PTX3 is produced at the actual site of inflammation.

PTX3 presents a low expression at normal conditions and may strongly increase under the induction of IL-1, IL-6, and TNF-α. Besides its importance as an inflammatory marker, PTX3 presents additional regulatory functions, including effects on angiogenesis, atherosclerotic lesion development, apoptotic cell clearance, tissue repair, and regulation of renal immunopathology [37]. As other inflammatory biomarkers, systemic levels of PTX3 also increase as renal function declines and predict increased cardiovascular and overall mortality risk in CKD patients, independent of traditional risk factors. Moreover, the finding that an inflammatory stimuli dramatically increase the expression of PTX3 in vascular endothelial cells suggested that PTX3 could be a useful marker for vascular pathology. However, further studies are needed to clarify the role of this inflammatory marker in CKD.

TNF-Like Weak Inducer of Apoptosis

Fibrosis is a major hallmark of progressive kidney disease. The cellular mechanisms that lead to kidney tissue fibrosis are complex and include increased inflammation, increased oxidative stress, and proximal tubule cell death in the form of apoptosis or senescence. Recent studies showed that TNF-like weak inducer of apoptosis (TWEAK) activates the fibroblast growth factor-inducible-14(Fn14) receptor, acting on intrinsic kidney cells and on inflammatory cells [38]. TWEAK induces the expression of inflammatory cytokines, downregulates the expression of klotho, is mitogenic, and in the presence of sensitizing agents promotes apoptosis. Its expression is increased in acute and chronic kidney injury and has been associated to higher mortality risk, especially when associated to systemic inflammation. CKD is a condition associated to klotho deficiency, which might contribute to accelerated aging, as klotho is an antiaging hormone with anti-inflammatory properties and highly expressed in kidney tubular cells. TWEAK reduces kidney klotho expression through NFκB activation and histone H3 and H4 deacetylation at the klotho promoter. Thus, TWEAK/Fn14 system promotes both NFκB-mediated activation of inflammation pathways and suppression of anti-inflammatory/antiaging pathways and is a potential player in inflammation-associated aging.

CKD Biomarkers and Anti-inflammatory Treatment Strategies

It becomes evident from the literature that a single biomarker is not sufficient to evaluate kidney disease stage, progression, and its associated cardiovascular risk. Due to the complexity of CKD and the coexistence of other pathological conditions, it is difficult to find a biomarker presenting all the characteristics of the ideal biomarker, which should be noninvasive (from readily available sources, as blood or urine); easily and rapidly measured, by using inexpensive and highly sensitive methods, allowing an early detection of the disease; and highly specific, being upregulated (or downregulated) specifically in case of the disease and not in case of coexistence of other pathological conditions; moreover, they should change rapidly in response to treatment and be useful in risk stratification and prognosis. Unfortunately, none of the traditional and newer biomarkers fulfill all these requisites.

There are several emergent biomarkers that need additional studies to establish their value as reliable biomarkers for CKD. These newer biomarkers may provide additional information about the local of predominant kidney damage and the underlying physiopathological mechanism of the disease; they may also be used as prognostic markers, evaluating if a patient is more likely to progress to ESKD and, therefore, if a more aggressive treatment is needed.

Recent data from the ongoing research showed that these promising disease-specific markers could be included in a panel of biomarkers for CKD that may supplement the more general markers of CKD. Indeed, as most of the studies are observational associations between biomarkers and outcomes, randomized trials are needed to evaluate the improvement in clinical outcome when using one biomarker or a panel of biomarkers to guide therapy or when interfering with the function of specific targeted biomarker(s).

Considering that circulating inflammatory markers are sensitive predictors of outcome in patients with CKD/ESKD, inflammation is believed to be a primary target for new therapeutic targeting in CKD.

After the exclusion of other complications that may underlie systemic inflammation, such as infections and dialysis modality-related causes, interventional strategies targeting persistent inflammation might be cautiously considered. Indeed, there is already scientific background for treatment of inflammation in CKD/ESKD; however, they have not been sufficiently powered by randomized clinical trials. A specific targeted anti-inflammatory approach with anticytokine therapies would have a beneficial impact beyond inflammation, on depression and fatigue that are often closely associated to inflammation in CKD. Antioxidant and antiwasting therapies may also contribute to modulate inflammation [39].

A biological treatment with etanercept, a TNF-α receptor antagonist, targeting uremic persistent inflammation was performed in a small number of patients on hemodialysis; after 44 weeks of treatment, etanercept showed positive effects on albumin and prealbumin levels, as compared to placebo, with no occurrence of adverse events; however, no significant changes were observed in CRP and IL-6. More promising results were observed for the treatment with recombinant human IL-1 receptor antagonist (IL-1ra). Actually, in a recent prospective controlled trial [40], 22 patients on hemodialysis, with increased markers of inflammation were randomized to recombinant human IL-1ra or placebo over 4 weeks. Patients who received IL-1ra treatment showed an impressive 53 % reduction in CRP, 40 % reduction in IL-6 levels and 23 % increase in mean prealbumin. Further studies are warranted to strength these results with IL-1ra treatment that may significantly improve protein-energy wasting and clinical outcomes.

Experimental and clinical evidence suggest a strong rationale for targeting IL-6 as a therapeutic strategy [41]. There are already some agents targeting IL-6 that are in clinical use or in preclinical studies. It has been reported that IL-6 may be a critical mediator in the pathophysiology of renal cancer and that high levels of IL-6 correlate with metastatic progression and poorer prognosis. In preclinical models, binding IL-6 resulted in tumor regression or prolonged survival.

IL-6 may activate cells through a conventional signaling, by linkage to the transmembrane receptor IL-6R expressed on the cell membrane, or by trans-signaling through the linkage of the complex soluble IL-6R/IL-6 to the membrane bound gp130, allowing the activation of cells lacking IL-6R. Siltuximab, an anti-IL-6 chimeric monoclonal antibody, and tocilizumab, a humanized anti-IL-6R monoclonal antibody, interfere with both classical and trans-signaling activation pathways.

Currently, siltuximab is already used to treat multiple myeloma and is under investigation in other malignancies, including renal cell carcinoma.

Renal cell carcinoma is a complication of acquired polycystic kidney disease, a condition associated with CKD that seems to be stimulated by renal inflammation. Siltuximab dose-ranging studies have been performed in renal cell carcinoma to assess the influence of this therapy, using CRP as the biomarker to monitor treatment. The first-in-human phase I/II study of siltuximab using continuous dosing in patients with metastatic renal cell carcinoma showed that, despite the low single-agent activity, the overall study results suggested the potential for further investigation of siltuximab either at higher doses and/or in combination with other active agents in the treatment of metastatic renal cell carcinoma [42].

Tocilizumab is licensed to treat rheumatoid arthritis and other inflammatory diseases. Some trials are studying the therapeutic potential of tocilizumab in CVD and the results may provide evidences suggesting a further therapeutic potential in CKD. Actually, there is little data concerning the use of biological therapy against IL-6 in renal diseases. Tocilizumab has been particularly used in patients with conditions where renal dysfunction was an associated comorbidity, namely, in lymphoproliferative disorders, AA amyloidosis, and Castleman's disease, and showed promising improvements in proteinuria and stabilization of renal function [43]. Definitive randomized controlled trials are, therefore, lacking in CKD.

As referred, the expression of sTWEAK and Fn14 is increased in acute and chronic kidney injury. Several studies showed that TWEAK has a deleterious role in kidney injury associated with inflammation through actions on intrinsic renal cells that include further promotion of inflammation and cell death. Currently, clinical trials exploring TWEAK/Fn14 targeting are ongoing in inflammatory disorders (rheumatoid arthritis, lupus nephritis) and cancer [38]. A phase I clinical trial with anti-TWEAK antibodies was recently completed in rheumatoid arthritis patients, who showed undetectable serum-TWEAK levels for up to 1 month as well as a trend toward decreased levels of several circulating biomarkers of systemic inflammation and no serious adverse effects were recorded. Moreover, a phase II randomized placebo-controlled clinical trial (ATLAS, Anti-Tweak in Lupus Nephritis Patients) is studying the efficacy, safety, and tolerability of the BIIB023 anti-TWEAK antibody as add-on therapy in class III/IV lupus nephritis patients who failed a complete remission within 3 months of initial therapy with steroids and mycophenolate mofetil. The primary outcome measure is the proportion of patients with complete and partial renal response from baseline to week 52. ATLAS was started in 2012 and the results are expected soon. Promising results from this clinical trial may expand the range of kidney disease in which TWEAK could be studied as a therapeutic target.

Another therapeutic approach is the modulation of inflammation through antioxidant agents, such as tocopherols and α-lipoic acid (ALA); however, the results from recent clinical trials have been controversial. A prospective [44], placebo-controlled, double-blind clinical trial studied 353 patients undergoing maintenance hemodialysis therapy, who were treated with oral antioxidant therapy over 6 months, and tested the impact on selected biomarkers of acute-phase inflammation, oxidative stress, and erythropoietic response; patients were randomly assigned to receive a combination of mixed tocopherols plus α-lipoic acid or matching placebos for 6 months; no major adverse events were observed, and both groups presented similar mortality and hospitalization rates along the study; the treatment with mixed tocopherols and ALA was generally safe and well tolerated but did not influence biomarkers of inflammation and oxidative stress or the erythropoietic response. Another randomized placebo-controlled trial [45] examined the effects of 2-month supplementation by vitamin E and ALA (alone or combined) on biomarkers of oxidative stress, inflammation, and malnutrition in 85 hemodialysis patients receiving ALA and vitamin E in mono- or combined therapy and found that inflammation and malnutrition status were improved, especially when treated with the combination of both, suggesting that this therapeutic approach might be useful as a preventive strategy against CVD in ESKD patients.

Considering that an inadequate dialyzer biocompatibility is still considered the most important cause of oxygen-free radical production during HD, the use of vitamin E-coated membrane dialyzers has been proposed as a strategy, based on the fact that vitamin E acts as a powerful hydrophilic scavenger, providing antioxidant protection to plasma lipids and cell membranes. A single-center, prospective, controlled, observational cohort study [46] evaluated the effects of vitamin E-coated membrane dialyzer on markers of oxidative stress and inflammation in 62 ESKD patients stabilized on standard chronic HD therapy for at least 6 months and found a significant reduction in inflammation and oxidative stress markers. These results suggest a potential beneficial effect from the long-term use of vitamin E-coated membranes; however, larger prospective randomized studies are warranted to strengthen these findings.

Statins are a well-established treatment for the primary and secondary prevention of atherosclerosis, reducing cardiovascular and all-cause mortality. Several studies showed that statins contribute also to decrease inflammatory cytokines; thus, statin therapy may be also beneficial in CKD/ESKD patients, by reducing inflammation. A systematic review of nine randomized controlled trials including 3,098 patients was recently performed to assess the effect of statins on chronic inflammation and nutrition status in dialysis patients [47]; this meta-analysis suggested that statins can improve the chronic inflammation status, whereas there is no conclusive evidence that it can improve the nutrition status. Considering that most of the included studies were small-scale single-center studies, most studies were not blinded, and some did not use a placebo in a control group and were heterogeneous with respect to treatment regimens and duration of follow-up, these findings need to be confirmed in well-designed and longer follow-up studies.

Concluding Remarks

In summary, there are several new promising biomarkers that might be used as a noninvasive tool in the diagnosis, prognosis, and management of various renal diseases. Most of these newer biomarkers can detect earlier renal injury, before serum creatinine, eGFR, and proteinuria increase. The reliance on only these traditional biomarkers may result in a long time lapse, along which successful interventions could be applied. Moreover, newer biomarkers, due to their specificity, can supplement traditional biomarkers by providing data about the physiopathological mechanism underlying the renal disease. The use of these biomarkers, as a noninvasive tool to study renal diseases, might be especially important in the pediatric age group, in whom the use of invasive investigation is a matter of concern.

It is unlikely that a single biomarker is able to predict CKD progression and cardiovascular morbidity and mortality, as well as to identify the multiple pathophysiological processes involved in CKD progression or in the underlying primary renal disease. Instead a panel of biomarkers will be more important for an earlier diagnosis and to access the outcome of the disease. Some of the reviewed biomarkers require further validation in enlarged clinical studies and others are already under study in clinical trials.

Acknowledgments/Support Authors thank the Portuguese Foundation for Science and Technology (FCT) , COMPETE-FEDER and POPH/FSE, through the following support: PTDC/SAU-TOX/114253/2009 and UID/NEU/04539/2013 (CNC.IBILI).

References

1. Fassett RG, Venuthurupalli SK, Gobe GC, Coombes JS, Cooper MA, Hoy WE. Biomarkers in chronic kidney disease: a review. Kidney Int. 2011;80:806–21.
2. Lenz O, Fornoni A. Chronic kidney disease care delivered by US family medicine and internal medicine trainees: results from an online survey. BMC Med. 2006;4:30–9.
3. KDIGO 2012. Clinical Practice Guideline for the Evaluation and Management of Chronic Kidney Disease. Chapter 2: Definition, identification, and prediction of CKD progression. Kidney Int. 2013;3(suppl):63–72.
4. Levin A, Rigatto C, Barrett B, Madore F, Muirhead N, Holmes D, Clase CM, Tang M, Djurdjev O, CanPREDDICT Investigators. Biomarkers of inflammation, fibrosis, cardiac stretch and injury predict death but not renal replacement therapy at 1 year in a Canadian chronic kidney disease cohort. Nephrol Dial Transplant. 2014;29:1037–47.
5. Junyent M, Martinez M, Borras M, et al. Usefulness of imaging techniques and novel biomarkers in the prediction of cardiovascular risk in patients with chronic kidney disease in Spain: the NEFRONA project. Nefrologia. 2010;30:119–26.
6. Fliser D, Kollerits B, Neyer U, et al. Fibroblast growth factor 23 (FGF23) predicts progression of chronic kidney disease: the Mild to Moderate Kidney Disease (MMKD) Study. J Am Soc Nephrol. 2007;18:2600–8.
7. Wheeler DC, Townend JN, Landray MJ. Cardiovascular risk factors in predialysis patients: baseline data from the Chronic Renal Impairment in Birmingham (CRIB) study. Kidney Int Suppl. 2003;84:S201–3.
8. Dajak M, Ignjatović S, Stojimirović B, Gajić S, Majkić-Singh N. Evaluation of renal damage by urinary beta-trace protein in patients with chronic kidney disease. Clin Lab. 2011;57:29–36.
9. Matsushita K, Sang Y, Ballew SH, Astor BC, Hoogeveen RC, Solomon SD, Ballantyne CM, Woodward M, Coresh J. Cardiac and kidney markers for cardiovascular prediction in individuals with chronic kidney disease: the Atherosclerosis Risk in Communities study. Arterioscler Thromb Vasc Biol. 2014;34:1770–7.
10. Bose B, Badve SV, Hiremath SS, Boudville N, Brown FG, Cass A, de Zoysa JR, Fassett RG, Faull R, Harris DC, Hawley CM, Kanellis J, Palmer SC, Perkovic V, Pascoe EM, Rangan GK,

Walker RJ, Walters G, Johnson DW. Effects of uric acid-lowering therapy on renal outcomes: a systematic review and meta-analysis. Nephrol Dial Transplant. 2014;29:406–13.

11. Liu KD, Yang W, Go AS, Anderson AH, Feldman HI, Fischer MJ, He J, Kallem RR, Kusek JW, Master SR, Miller ER 3rd, Rosas SE, Steigerwalt S, Tao K, Weir MR, Hsu CY; CRIC Study Investigators. Urine neutrophil gelatinase-associated lipocalin and risk of cardiovascular disease and death in CKD: results from the Chronic Renal Insufficiency Cohort (CRIC) Study. Am J Kidney Dis. 2015; 65(2):267–74.
12. Peralta CA, Katz R, Bonventre JV, Sabbisetti V, Siscovick D, Sarnak M, Shlipak MG. Associations of urinary levels of kidney injury molecule 1 (KIM-1) and neutrophil gelatinase-associated lipocalin (NGAL) with kidney function decline in the Multi-Ethnic Study of Atherosclerosis (MESA). Am J Kidney Dis. 2012;60:904–11.
13. van Timmeren MM, Vaidya VS, van Ree RM, et al. High urinary excretion of kidney injury molecule-1 is an independent predictor of graft loss in renal transplant recipients. Transplantation. 2007;84:1625–30.
14. Cowland JB, Borregaard N. Molecular characterization and pattern of tissue expression of the gene for neutrophil gelatinase-associated lipocalin from humans. Genomics. 1997;45:17–23.
15. Haase M, Devarajan P, Haase-Fielitz A, Bellomo R, Cruz DN, Wagener G, et al. The outcome of neutrophil gelatinase-associated lipocalin (NGAL)-positive subclinical acute kidney injury: a multicenter pooled analysis of prospective studies. J Am Coll Cardiol. 2011;57:1752–61.
16. Kamijo-Ikemori A, Sugaya T, Ichikawa D, Hoshino S, Matsui K, Yokoyama T, Yasuda T, Hirata K, Kimura K. Urinary liver type fatty acid binding protein in diabetic nephropathy. Clin Chim Acta. 2013;424:104–8.
17. Kamijo A, Sugaya T, Hikawa A, Yamanouchi M, Hirata Y, Ishimitsu T, Numabe A, Takagi M, Hayakawa H, Tabei F, Sugimoto T, Mise N, Omata M, Kimura K. Urinary liver-type fatty acid binding protein as a useful biomarker in chronic kidney disease. Mol Cell Biochem. 2006;284:175–82.
18. Yang J, Choi HM, Seo MY, Lee JY, Kim K, Jun H, Jung CW, Park KT, Kim MG, Jo SK, Cho W, Kim HK. Urine liver-type fatty acid-binding protein predicts graft outcome up to 2 years after kidney transplantation. Transplant Proc. 2014;46:376–80.
19. Hörstrup JH, Gehrmann M, Schneider B, Plöger A, Froese P, Schirop T, Kampf D, Frei U, Neumann R, Eckardt KU. Elevation of serum and urine levels of TIMP-1 and tenascin in patients with renal disease. Nephrol Dial Transplant. 2002;17:1005–13.
20. Hanamura K, Tojo A, Fujita T. Urinary and glomerular podocytes in patients with chronic kidney diseases. Clin Exp Nephrol. 2014;18:95–103.
21. Zoccali C, Bode-Böger SM, Mallamaci F, Benedetto FA, Tripepi G, Malatino LS, Cataliotti A, Bellanuova I, Fermo I, Frölich JC, Böger RH. Plasma concentration of asymmetrical dimethylarginine and mortality in patients with end-stage renal disease: a prospective study. Lancet. 2001;358:2113–7.
22. Raptis V, Kapoulas S, Grekas D. Role of asymmetrical dimethylarginine in the progression of renal disease. Nephrology. 2013;18:11–21.
23. Sibal L, Agarwal SC, Home PD, Boger RH. The role of asymmetric dimethylarginine (ADMA) in endothelial dysfunction and cardiovascular disease. Curr Cardiol Rev. 2010;6:82–90.
24. Eiselta J, Rajdlb D, Racekb J, Vostrýb M, Rulcováa K, Wirtha J. Asymmetric dimethylarginine and progression of chronic kidney disease – a one-year follow-up study. Kidney Blood Press Res. 2014;39:50–7.
25. Eddy AA. Proteinuria and interstitial injury. Nephrol Dial Transplant. 2004;19:277–81.
26. Costa E, Lima M, Alves JM, Rocha S, Rocha-Pereira P, Castro E, Miranda V, Faria MS, Loureiro A, Quintanilha A, Belo L, Santos-Silva A. Inflammation, T-cell phenotype, and inflammatory cytokines in chronic kidney disease patients under hemodialysis and its relationship to resistance to recombinant human erythropoietin therapy. J Clin Immunol. 2008;28:268–75.
27. Fried L, Solomon C, Shlipak M, et al. Inflammatory and prothrombotic markers and the progression of renal disease in elderly individuals. J Am Soc Nephrol. 2004;15:3184–91.

28. Keller C, Katz R, Cushman M, et al. Association of kidney function with inflammatory and procoagulant markers in a diverse cohort: a cross-sectional analysis from the Multi-Ethnic Study of Atherosclerosis (MESA). BMC Nephrol. 2008;9:9.
29. Tonelli M, Sacks F, Pfeffer M, et al. Biomarkers of inflammation and progression of chronic kidney disease. Kidney Int. 2005;68:237–45.
30. Lin J, Hu FB, Rimm EB, et al. The association of serum lipids and inflammatory biomarkers with renal function in men with type II diabetes mellitus. Kidney Int. 2006;69:336–42.
31. Mallamaci F, Tripepi G, Cutrupi S, et al. Prognostic value of combined use of biomarkers of inflammation, endothelial dysfunction, and myocardiopathy in patients with ESRD. Kidney Int. 2005;67:2330–7.
32. Menon V, Greene T, Wang X, et al. C-reactive protein and albumin as predictors of all-cause and cardiovascular mortality in chronic kidney disease. Kidney Int. 2005;68:766–72.
33. Go AS, Chertow GM, Fan D, et al. Chronic kidney disease and the risks of death, cardiovascular events, and hospitalization. N Engl J Med. 2004;351:1296–305.
34. Upadhyay A, Larson MG, Guo C-Y, Vasan RS, Lipinska I, O'Donnell CJ, Kathiresan S, Meigs JB, Keaney Jr JF, Rong J, Benjamin EJ, Fox CS. Inflammation, kidney function and albuminuria in the Framingham Offspring cohort. Nephrol Dial Transplant. 2011;26:920–6.
35. Kawaguchi T, Tong L, Robinson BM, Sen A, Fukuhara S, Kurokawa K, Canaud B, Lameire N, Port FK, Pisoni RL. C-reactive protein and mortality in hemodialysis patients: the Dialysis Outcomes and Practice Patterns Study (DOPPS). Nephron Clin Pract. 2011;117:c167–78.
36. Carrero JJ, Stenvinkel P. Inflammation in end-stage renal disease – what have we learned in 10 years? Semin Dial. 2010;23:498–509.
37. Witasp A, Rydén M, Carrero JJ, Qureshi AR, Nordfors L, Näslund E, Hammarqvist F, Arefin S, Kublickiene K, Stenvinkel P. Elevated circulating levels and tissue expression of pentraxin 3 in uremia: a reflection of endothelial dysfunction. PLoS One. 2013;8(5):e63493.
38. Sanz AB, Izquierdo MC, Sanchez-Niño MD, Ucero AC, Egido J, Ruiz-Ortega M, Ramos AM, Putterman C, Ortiz A. TWEAK and the progression of renal disease: clinical translation. Nephrol Dial Transplant. 2014;29 Suppl 1:i54–62.
39. Miyamoto T, Carrero JJ, Stenvinkelb P. Inflammation as a risk factor and target for therapy in chronic kidney disease. Curr Opin Nephrol Hypertens. 2011;20:662–8.
40. Hung AM, Ellis CD, Shintani A, Booker C, Ikizler TA. IL-1b receptor antagonist reduces inflammation in hemodialysis patients. J Am Soc Nephrol. 2011;22:437–42.
41. Puchalski T, Prabhakar U, Jiao Q, Berns B, Davis HM. Pharmacokinetic and pharmacodynamic modeling of an anti-interleukin-6 chimeric monoclonal antibody (siltuximab) in patients with metastatic renal cell carcinoma. Clin Cancer Res. 2010;16:1652–61.
42. Rossi JF, Négrier S, James ND, Kocak I, Hawkins R, Davis H, Prabhakar U, Qin X, Mulders P, Berns B. A phase I/II study of siltuximab (CNTO 328), an anti-interleukin-6 monoclonal antibody, in metastatic renal cell cancer. Br J Cancer. 2010;103:1154–62.
43. Jones SA, Fraser DJ, Fielding CA, Jones GW. Interleukin 6 in renal disease and therapy. Nephrol Dial Transplant. 2014. http://ndt.oxfordjournals.org/content/early/2014/07/09/ndt.gfu233.full.pdf+html.
44. Himmelfarb J, Ikizler TA, Ellis C, Wu P, Shintani A, Dalal S, Kaplan M, Chonchol M, Hakim RM. Provision of antioxidant therapy in hemodialysis (PATH): a randomized clinical trial. J Am Soc Nephrol. 2014;25:623–33.
45. Ahmadi A, Mazooji N, Roozbeh J, Mazloom Z, Hasanzade J. Effect of alpha-lipoic acid and vitamin E supplementation on oxidative stress, inflammation, and malnutrition in hemodialysis patients. Iran J Kidney Dis. 2013;7:461–7.
46. Kirmizis D, Papagianni A, Belechri AM, Memmos D. Effects of vitamin E-coated membrane dialyser on markers of oxidative stress and inflammation in patients on chronic haemodialysis. Nephrol Dial Transplant. 2011;26:2296–301.
47. Deng J, Wu Q, Liao Y, Huo D, Yang Z. Effect of statins on chronic inflammation and nutrition status in renal dialysis patients: a systematic review and meta-analysis. Nephrology. 2012;17:545–51.

Chapter 6
Immune-Mediated Inflammatory Rheumatic Diseases

Maria José Santos, Ana Cristina Cordeiro, and Victor M. Gil

Abstract Atherosclerosis occurs earlier and progresses more rapidly in patients with immune-mediated inflammatory rheumatic disorders. Cardiovascular (CV) disease is the leading cause of death in this context, and the relative risk for CV events is strikingly high, especially among young women. This excessive risk is not fully explained by traditional CV risk factors, and the disease itself is of paramount relevance. Systemic inflammation enhances atherogenesis throughout the whole process. Circulating inflammatory cytokines foster early vascular dysfunction as well as subclinical structural lesions, plaque rupture and thrombosis. Several biomarkers of atherosclerosis have been identified in rheumatic diseases. With few exceptions, their applicability in clinical practice is still marginal.

Keywords Rheumatic diseases • Autoimmunity • Inflammation • Autoantibodies • Atherosclerosis

It has been recognized for decades now that patients with immune-mediated inflammatory disorders experience cardiovascular (CV) events more often than their age- and gender-matched counterparts and are at increased risk of death from CV diseases. In addition, a significant proportion of these patients evidence premature subclinical vascular disease, including impaired endothelial function, increased intima-media thickness (IMT), increased arterial stiffness, higher prevalence of atherosclerotic plaques, myocardial perfusion abnormalities or increased coronary artery calcium (CAC) score. Chronic inflammation has been suggested as an important contributor to premature vascular damage in this context.

Immune-mediated rheumatic diseases represent a heterogeneous group of disorders where the production of autoantibodies and chronic inflammation often coexist.

M.J. Santos, M.D., Ph.D. (✉) • A.C. Cordeiro, M.D.
Department of Rheumatology, Hospital Garcia de Orta,
Avenida Prof. Torrado da Silva, 2801-951 Almada, Portugal
e-mail: mjps1234@gmail.com

V.M. Gil, M.D., Ph.D.
Department of Cardiology, Hospital dos Lusíadas, Lisbon, Portugal

© Springer International Publishing Switzerland 2015
F. Palavra et al. (eds.), *Biomarkers of Cardiometabolic Risk, Inflammation and Disease*, DOI 10.1007/978-3-319-16018-4_6

Table 6.1 The relative risk of incident MI and stroke in SLE [5], RA [6], SSc [7], systemic vasculitis [10, 12] and pSS [11]: results from systematic literature reviews, meta-analysis and population-based reports

	MI	Stroke
	Risk ratio (95 % CI)	Risk ratio (95 % CI)
SLE	2.25 (1.37–3.68)	2.29 (0.85–6.15)
RA	2.10 (1.52–2.89)	1.91 (1.73–2.12)
SSc	1.82 (1.40–2.36)	1.43 (1.12–1.83)
Systemic vasculitis	2.50 (1.60–3.70)[a]	
	0.74 (0.44, 1.26)[b]	1.40 (0.60–3.30)[c]
pSS	2.40 (1.50–3.80)	1.60 (1.00–2.80)

MI myocardial infarction, *SLE* systemic lupus erythematosus, *RA* rheumatoid arthritis, *SSc* systemic sclerosis, *pSS* primary Sjögren's syndrome

[a]Observed/estimated risk of MI in Wegener's granulomatosis

[b]HR of MI in giant cell arteritis

[c]Incidence rate ratio of stoke within the 2 years following diagnosis of giant cell arteritis

Several epidemiological studies demonstrated that CV diseases are among the leading cause of death in systemic lupus erythematosus (SLE) [1] and in rheumatoid arthritis (RA) patients [2], and despite all the advances in management of these diseases that resulted in an overall better prognosis, CV mortality did not improve throughout the last decades. As consequence, the CV mortality gap between patients and the general population has widened [3]. SLE and RA are associated with an increased risk for ischemic heart disease, congestive heart failure and stroke especially in younger ages [4–6]. More recently, this increased CV risk has been also demonstrated for other rheumatic diseases, including systemic sclerosis (SSc) [7, 8], systemic vasculitis [9, 10] and primary Sjögren's syndrome (pSS) (Table 6.1) [11].

In comparison with the general population, atherosclerosis occurs earlier and progresses more rapidly in immune-mediated inflammatory rheumatic diseases. The chronological age of the patients is not concordant with the state of their arteries, which are ageing prematurely. The mechanisms underlying accelerated atherosclerosis are complex and represent an area of intense investigation. Systemic rheumatic diseases can be a useful model to expand the understanding of mechanisms behind atherogenesis.

Although traditional cardiovascular risk factors predict CV outcomes, they do not fully explain the excessive risk observed in patients suffering from inflammatory rheumatic diseases. Competing risks such as the disease itself and disease-specific factors, including chronic inflammation, vasculopathic changes and also the effect of medication, are among the most widely accepted hypothesis. It has been suggested that despite the overall increased risk, the relative contribution of traditional CV risk factors might be smaller due to the presence of those competing risks [12, 13].

Systemic Inflammation as the Main Driver of Cardiovascular Risk in Rheumatic Diseases

The atherosclerotic process begins early in life with the accumulation of lipid-laden cells beneath the endothelium – the fatty streak – that includes mainly macrophages and some T cells. The fatty streak can vanish or may progress to atheroma formation. Atheromata consist of cells, connective tissue elements, lipids and debris that together thicken the intima. Inflammatory and immune cells constitute an important part of the atherosclerotic lesions. LDL cholesterol infiltrates the wall of large- and medium-sized arteries where it is responsible for initiating an inflammatory response. LDL oxidation evokes the release of phospholipids that activate the endothelium mainly at sites of hemodynamic strain (high oscillatory, but low average shear stress), which leads to increased expression of adhesion molecules and inflammatory cytokines. Blood platelets adhere to surface molecules of endothelial cells via their glycoproteins IIb/IIIa.

The atheroma possesses a central core with foam cells and extracellular lipid droplets surrounded by a cap of smooth muscle cells and a collagen-rich matrix. Atheroma growing involves infiltration by T cells, macrophages and mast cells; many of them are activated and produce pro-inflammatory cytokines (interleukin-1β, tumour necrosis factor, γ-interferon) that promote the migration and proliferation of smooth muscle cells and the construction of a dense extracellular matrix – the advance atherosclerotic lesion.

The acute coronary syndromes are usually initiated by a rupture of the fibrous cap but in some cases can occur just by endothelial erosion. In one quarter of cases, the endothelium does not rupture, but instead it is replaced for prothrombotic inflammatory cells. Plaque rupture usually occurs in areas of sustained inflammation, macrophage accumulation and apoptosis. Proteolytic enzymes produced by activated macrophages can degrade the collagen of the fibrous cap facilitating its rupture. These enzymes belong to the matrix metalloproteinase (MMP) family. The three MMPs [1, 8, 13] are overproduced by macrophages present in lesions where massive thrombosis has occurred. Furthermore, it seems to be a crosstalk between this immune effector macrophage pathway and adaptive immune cells (T cells) inhibiting the synthesis and augmenting the degradation of interstitial collagen. In fact, it has been demonstrated that T-cell-derived cytokine CD40 ligand (CD154) boosts the production of interstitial collagenase by human macrophages.

The observations above provide a cellular and molecular mechanism linking inflammation to the thinning and weakening of the fibrous cap, which can precipitate plaque rupture, thrombosis and acute CV events. Longitudinal studies have demonstrated that the overall disease activity, a proxy of inflammatory burden, is crucial for cardiovascular outcome of immune-mediated inflammatory rheumatic diseases [14]. Steiman et al. showed in SLE patients the predictive value of disease activity by demonstrating that clinically active lupus patients are at higher CV risk than serologically active clinically quiescent patients. After a 10-year follow-up, 7.3 % of clinically active patients developed new coronary events comparing to

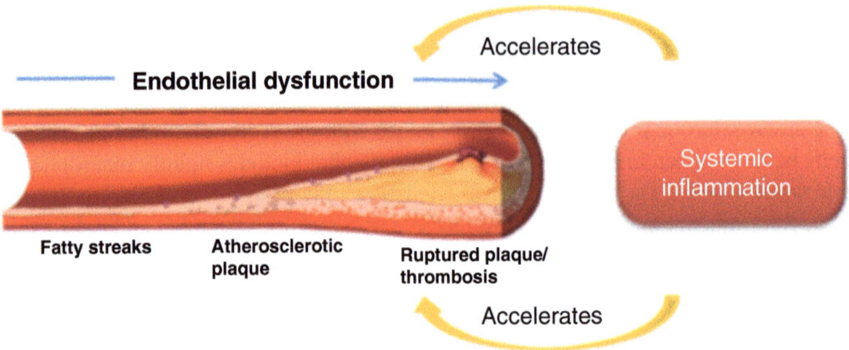

Fig. 6.1 The interplay of systemic inflammation and atherosclerosis progression

1.8 % of those with clinically quiescent disease [15]. Likewise, in RA patients, systemic inflammation and CV risk factors predict greater IMT progression rate [16]. High levels of inflammatory cytokines generate a spectrum of pro-atherogenic changes that fosters atherosclerosis development and progression. A direct effect on the vasculature can be observed throughout the whole process, that is, from early endothelial dysfunction to plaque rupture and the occurrence of a thrombotic event (Fig. 6.1). Not only endothelial function and repair are negatively affected by increased circulating levels of pro-inflammatory cytokines such as tumour necrosis factor (TNF), interleukin (IL)-Iβ or IL-6 but also high levels of inflammation are associated with plaque instability and rupture.

In addition, systemic inflammation affects several other pathways through which may contribute to accelerated atherogenesis:

- Insulin resistance
- Dyslipidaemia
- Prothrombotic status
- Oxidative stress
- Abnormal body composition phenotype

The association between inflammatory biomarkers and the risk for future CV events has been recognized in several clinical and epidemiological observations. While high levels of C-reactive protein (CRP) are present in major inflammatory situations, high-sensitivity (hs) CRP elevation coexists with states of low-grade inflammation such as atherosclerosis. CRP has been associated with a number of CV risk factors like obesity, smoking, heart rate, high blood pressure, high serum fibrinogen, hypercholesterolaemia, hypertriglyceridaemia, apolipoprotein B or increased fasting blood glucose. In the general population, hsCRP is an independent predictor of future vascular events at any level of LDL cholesterol and, in association with LDL cholesterol levels, it improves the individual estimation of CV risk.

Nonetheless, in patients with rheumatic diseases, where highly increased CRP is a characteristic, the relationship of this inflammatory biomarker to subsequent clinical events has not been consistently established.

Endothelial Activation and Dysfunction

Endothelial cells (EC) are crucial in maintaining blood fluidity and in regulating vascular tonus and permeability. Under normal conditions, EC express molecules that prevent platelet aggregation and clot formation. Inflammatory cytokines modify endothelial homeostasis that results in increased expression of adhesion molecules, loss of antithrombotic properties, increased permeability and reduced ability to produce NO in response to several stimuli. Intercellular adhesion molecules and chemokines mediate leukocyte adhesion to endothelial cells or extracellular matrix, endothelial transmigration and leukocyte activation. Endothelial activation and dysfunction are chief phenomena in early atherogenesis and precedes structural vascular changes. Endothelial dysfunction is potentially reversible with the control of the underlying inflammatory condition.

Along with non-invasive endothelial function testing (e.g. endothelium-dependent flow-mediated dilation, peripheral artery tonometry, pulse wave velocity measurement), circulating biomarkers of endothelial activation have been studied in systemic rheumatic diseases. Increased levels of E-selectin, sICAM-1, VCAM, thrombomodulin (TM) and tissue factor (TF) were identified in relation to disease activity [17].

Another surrogate marker of EC function is the number of circulating endothelial progenitor cells (EPC) and endothelial microparticles. EPC are a heterogeneous cell population derived from the bone marrow involved in angiogenesis and repair of endothelium. Variations in the level of circulating and mature EPC or EPC impaired function have been documented in active RA, SLE and pSS, suggesting compromised endothelial repair [18, 19].

Inflammation and Atherothrombosis

The progression of atherosclerosis and local thrombosis is closely linked phenomena that may culminate in a thrombotic occlusion of the vascular lumen and consequent acute CV event. Alterations of haemostatic and haemorheologic factors contribute to atherogenesis and are related to vascular ischemic events in the general population [20].

In immune-mediated inflammatory rheumatic diseases, both altered blood rheology and high levels of haemostatic biomarkers have been found in association with subclinical atherosclerosis [21]. Serum levels of haemostatic factors, namely, von Willebrand factor (vWF), plasminogen activator inhibitor (PAI)-1, thrombomodulin and tissue factor, are related to inflammatory status. Some of these markers (PAI-1 and vWF) were studied in RA patients and baseline values found to be independent predictors of future CV events.

Patients have reduced erythrocyte deformability and increased erythrocyte aggregation, which may contribute to impaired microcirculation and microvascular dysfunction. The interaction between inflammation and thrombogenesis is not entirely understood. Nevertheless, we and others found disturbed and unfavourable haemorheologic phenotype in association with active RA and active SLE, and this might represent an additional link between inflammation and atherogenesis [21].

Autoantibodies

The contribution of autoantibodies to atherogenesis remains unclear in the scope of rheumatic diseases, yet the current evidence suggests a relationship between some autoantibodies and subclinical atherosclerosis. Increased production of anti-endothelial cell antibodies, a putative marker of vascular damage, has been reported in SLE, RA, systemic vasculitis and other rheumatic diseases [22]. Oxidation is one of the major aspects involved in atheroma development, and high levels of antibodies against oxidized low-density lipoproteins (ox-LDL), a quantifiable marker of oxidative stress present over a certain time period, are found in a significant proportion of lupus patients [23], although their biological role is not well established.

Antiphospholipid antibodies, a family of autoantibodies directed against phospholipid-binding plasma proteins, are strongly associated with thrombosis and pregnancy morbidity. Anti-cardiolipin (aCl) and anti-β2 glycoprotein I antibodies are the most extensively studied, but other antiphospholipid (aPL) antibodies are implicated in CV events through thrombotic pathways. It has been hypothesized that non-thrombotic mechanisms might also relate aPL and CV events. A possible mechanism linking aPL and atherogenesis is their role in inducing oxidative stress. Moreover, anti-cardiolipin antibodies directly interfere with paraoxonase activity, a high-density lipoprotein-related antioxidant enzyme, adding to the oxidative stress found in these conditions [24]. In fact, some small studies found an association between aPL titres and features of subclinical atherosclerosis (increased IMT and CAC score). Furthermore, low levels of IgM anti-oxidized cardiolipin and anti-oxidized phosphatidylserine were found more frequently in lupus patients with carotid plaques compared to those without plaques [25]. More recently, the presence of aPL was shown to be predictive of CAC score > 0 at 15 and 20 years in the large Coronary Artery Risk Development in Young Adults (CARDIA) cohort [26].

Control of Inflammation and CV Risk

Evidence shows that treatment of inflammation reduces CV burden related to systemic rheumatic diseases. The effective control of disease activity can revert early vascular changes measured by endothelium-dependent flow-mediated dilation (FMD), prevent progression of subclinical atherosclerosis and more importantly reduce incident CV events and CV death. Methotrexate is a disease-modifier anti-rheumatic drug (DMARD) broadly used for the treatment of chronic inflammatory rheumatic disorders. There is substantial documentation that its use not only controls arthritis and improves disease-specific outcomes but significantly reduces the risk of CV events and death in RA patients [27]. A recent meta-analysis reports a 21 % lower risk for fatal and nonfatal hard CV events in methotrexate users (RA, psoriasis and polyarthritis) after a median follow-up of 5.84 years (relative risk 0.79; 95 % CI 0.73–0.87), and risk reduction was even greater when analysis was adjusted for disease activity [28]. More recently, the introduction of biological therapies revolutionized the control of clinical manifestations and of structural damage progression in an important proportion of patients who failed synthetic DMARDs. Inhibition of TNF, available for the last 15 years, is associated with improvement of endothelial function [29], prevention of atherosclerosis progression [30] and reduction of risk for all cardiovascular events [31]. The impact of biologics with other mode of action remains largely unknown, although improvement of endothelial function was documented in the short term after IL-6 blockade.

Other antirheumatic medications may also have a beneficial effect on atherogenesis, but except for antimalarials, data is limited. The use of hydroxychloroquine is associated with reduced risk of subclinical atherosclerosis, CV events and overall mortality in lupus patients, but the mechanisms underlying this benefit remain largely undetermined.

The debate around the effect of corticosteroids in atherogenesis continues. If on the one hand corticosteroids have a potent anti-inflammatory effect, on the other hand, this group of drugs has a negative impact on CV risk factors, including weight gain, worsening insulin resistance, hypertension and hyperlipidaemia. Thus, the balance between risk and benefit depends on corticosteroid dosage and duration of treatment.

The Examples of Systemic Rheumatic Diseases

Rheumatoid Arthritis

Rheumatoid arthritis (RA) is the prototype of chronic inflammatory arthropathy that affects 0.5–1 % of the adult world population. Several studies, mainly from Europe, have clearly demonstrated that patients with RA have reduced life expectancy largely as a consequence of an excess of CV deaths. In a recent review of CV comorbidity in rheumatic diseases, Symmons et al. report the results of a meta-analysis of 24 mortality studies in RA published between 1970 and 2005 showing a weighted combined all-cause standardized mortality ratio (met-SMR) of 1.50 (95 % 1.39–1.61) with similar increases for IHD (met-SMR 1.59; 95 %CI 1.46–1.73) and stroke (met-SMR 1.52; 95 % CI 1.40–1.67) [13]. The excess of CV deaths is not apparent at disease onset; it is rather a feature of established RA, positive for rheumatoid factor. Besides fatal events, the risk of nonfatal myocardial infarction (MI) and stroke is about two times higher in RA compared to sex- and age-matched controls [6]. Similarly, subclinical atherosclerosis is identified more frequently in rheumatoid arthritis. Carotid ultrasound is an easy to perform non-invasive method to assess the presence of plaques and the intima-media thickness (IMT). Carotid and coronary atheroscleroses are highly correlated and independent predictors of CV events. A significantly higher prevalence of carotid plaques was shown in RA in comparison with sex-, age- and ethnicity-matched controls (44 % vs 15 %; $p<0.001$) [32].

Concerning carotid IMT, results are controversial, and not all studies have established an association between greater IMT in RA diagnosis [32]. IMT correlates with the presence of traditional CV risk factors, but it seems to be a less robust predictor of CV events. Coronary artery calcium (CAC) is another surrogate marker of atherosclerosis that helps CV risk stratification in the general population. The prevalence and the extent of CAC is larger in RA (47.6 %) than in controls (35.2 %) [33]. Macrovascular and microvascular functions are frequently impaired in parallel with disease activity. Using brachial artery FMD, many groups have shown impaired endothelial function in RA. Endothelial dysfunction is related to disease activity and reverts with the treatment of active RA.

Traditional CV Risk Factors

The burden of traditional CV risk factors is high in RA. Hypertension affects more than 40 % of patients, and although its overall prevalence is similar in RA and controls, evidence suggests it may be higher in younger patients and linked to active disease. The inflammatory process affects not only lipid concentration but also function. Dyslipidemia is common and correlates with disease activity. Lipid alterations, mainly reduced HDL cholesterol and increased triglycerides, are present in about half of the patients and may precede the diagnosis of RA. Inflammation alters HDL structure, and HDL loses its anti-inflammatory, antioxidant and cardioprotective properties and may become pro-inflammatory (piHDL). Also insulin resistance and diabetes have been consistently reported more frequently in RA.

Nontraditional Biomarkers

Biomarkers of endothelial activation (VCAM-1 and ICAM-1) are elevated in RA patients and correlate with subclinical atherosclerosis. IL-6 is more strongly associated with endothelial dysfunction than CRP or ESR.

In line with longitudinal studies in the general population, haemostatic factors PAI-1 and vWF were found to be strongly predictive of new CV events in established RA. Also serum levels of asymmetric dimethylarginine (ADMA) are elevated in untreated early arthritis and have a negative effect in coronary flow reserve. After treatment of arthritis, ADMA concentration decreases.

As expected, RA patients have higher levels of inflammatory biomarkers than controls. Some studies, but not all, found increased levels of CRP, IL-1, IL-6 and TNF to be associated with impaired FMD and increased IMT [34].

Many other surrogate markers of endothelial activation, including MCP-1, adiponectin, have been studied in RA as potential biomarkers of atherosclerosis. Nevertheless, the cross-sectional design of most studies, the limited number of participants and the heterogeneity of the endpoints hamper definitive conclusions regarding the reported associations.

RA Medication

As stated before, the control of inflammation has documented benefit on atherogenesis. The use of methotrexate and of biologics decreases CV risk. The benefit was demonstrated not only for subclinical disease but also most importantly the reduction of CV events and also mortality was recognized. On the other side, the use of NSAIDs and corticosteroids aggravates some traditional CV risk factors.

Systemic Lupus Erythematosus

Systemic lupus erythematosus (SLE) is a multiorgan disease characterized by the production of autoantibodies with an estimated prevalence of 70–110/100,000 inhabitants in South European countries. SLE affects preferentially women of reproductive age and has a mortality risk of over three times that of the population. The higher proportion of deaths beyond 5 years of diagnosis is attributable to atherosclerosis. The prevalence of premature atherosclerosis is remarkable in young females. Most studies report a two- to tenfold increase in the risk of MI among SLE patients, although the relative risk may be as high as 52-fold in women with lupus aged 35–44 years [35]. SLE patients have also increase risk of congestive heart failure and stoke. Again, the relative risk of cerebrovascular disease is higher among premenopausal women. Many studies addressed subclinical atherosclerosis and consistently documented higher prevalence of carotid plaques and CAC score. Regarding cIMT, it is not clear whether it is increased or not. While some groups found greater cIMT, others found no difference between lupus patients and controls.

Endothelial dysfunction, assessed by FMD, is an early event frequently reported among patients with SLE.

Substantial amount of research has focused on the identification of risk factors, and similar to RA, traditional CV risk factors and disease-related and treatment-related factors all have been associated with premature atherosclerosis in lupus.

Traditional cardiovascular risk factors are highly prevalent in SLE. Hypertension was reported in 33 % of SLE patients from the Toronto Lupus Cohort compared to 13 % of age-matched controls. Hypertension is associated with a one- to twofold increased risk of coronary artery disease. Hypercholesterolemia is common and likewise associated with increased risk for CV events. Older age and male gender are also predictors of CV events in lupus. The risk for CV events is four times higher in male patients compared to females.

Nontraditional Biomarkers

Contrasting to the general population where hsCRP is a predictor of subsequent CV events and reflects subclinical inflammation, this association is less consistent in lupus patients. Nevertheless, in the LUMINA cohort, elevated CRP was associated with increased CV risk, and another study also found high hsCRP (above 1.6 mg/l) associated with a HR 3.37 for MI and angina.

Pro-inflammatory HDL (piHDL) can be detected in up to 45 % of SLE patients and correlates with cIMT and carotid plaques.

Some autoantibodies have been considered as possible predictors of atherosclerosis. Antiphospholipid antibodies are found in approximately one-third of lupus patients. The positivity for aPL presents a four-time higher risk of having MI, stroke or peripheral vascular disease. Along with increased risk for both arterial and venous thrombosis, there is some evidence linking aPL and carotid IMT. aPLs were described as stimulators of tissue factor (TF) expression on the surface of peripheral blood mononuclear cells, and given the role of TF in atherothrombosis, it was postulated that TF may play a role in lupus CV disease.

A recent study found that defensins are elevated in lupus patients and are predictive of future CV events and subclinical atherosclerosis.

SLE disease itself emerged as an important CV risk, and higher SLE disease activity measured by the SLEDAI was predictive of future CV events in some cohort studies.

SLE Medication

Corticosteroids remain the cornerstone treatment for severe lupus. Their side effects are well established and include the worsening of some traditional CV risk factors. Nevertheless, by controlling disease activity may counteract some negative effects on the vascular system. The effect of corticosteroids on CV disease remains controversial, and probably the relationship is not linear.

On the contrary, the vasculoprotective effect of antimalarials is now well recognized.

Immunosuppressants such as mycophenolate mofetil and cyclophosphamide are likely to reduce CV burden.

The effect of statins was studied in SLE patients without CV events with surprising negative results. Although cholesterol levels diminished, no effect could be demonstrated on markers of endothelial activation, disease activity or measures of subclinical atherosclerosis. Changes in CAC score and IMT at 2 years were similar in the treated and in the placebo group.

Systemic Sclerosis

Systemic sclerosis (SSc) is a multisystem disease characterized by vascular inflammation, vascular hyperactivity and excess tissue collagen deposition that leads to fibrosis of the skin and internal organs [36, 37]. It affects both the macrocirculation and the microcirculation [38, 39] with an accelerated injury to the vessel wall.

The exact mechanism and triggers for endothelial dysfunction with endothelial cell activation and altered vascular tone are still unclear, but several mediators, loss of redox control and hypoxia [39] contribute to the perpetuation of the pathologic changes. Similarly to other connective tissue diseases, SSc patients have been found to be prone to accelerated atherosclerosis and increased coronary artery disease, with increased morbidity and mortality [40] not fully explained by traditional Framingham cardiovascular risk factors.

Despite recognized vascular involvement in SSc, there is a paucity of robust data regarding cardiovascular, coronary disease and atherosclerosis in large SSc cohorts. Recent clinical databases estimate however that around 29 % of mortality in SSc is due to CV causes [40]. Also, recent published data estimates that around 5.4 % of SSc patients' hospitalizations in the USA are associated with atherosclerotic cardiovascular disease with a higher in-hospital mortality rate compared to patients with RA and SLE [41].

Cardiac involvement in SSc is estimated around 25 % and comprises manifestations of all heart structures including congestive heart failure, pericardial effusion, conduction disturbances and coronary artery disease. Contraction band myocardial necrosis resulting from ischemia and myocardial fibrosis is the most common pathological finding [42].

In terms of coronary heart disease (CHD), two studies demonstrated that SSc has a higher risk of CHD (two- to threefold increase) and is associated with an increased risk of myocardial infarction compared to general population [43] and that the risk for CHD remains, even after the adjustment to traditional CV risk factors [44]. The underlying mechanisms may be related to positive aPL, coronary stenosis, coronary ectasia, slow flow, vessel tortuosity, calcification and spasm [45].

Very few studies addressing cerebrovascular disease have been published in SSc and with conflicting results. One study showed no apparent difference in the prevalence of atherosclerosis comparing to general population; another demonstrated carotid artery stenosis by colour Doppler ultrasound in 64 % of patients [46], and another one demonstrated a higher prevalence of carotid plaque in SSc patients compared to matched controls [47].

The most studied and feared vascular damage in SSc is related to pulmonary arterial hypertension (PAH), one of the leading mortality causes in SSc. A mean pulmonary pressure greater than 25 mmHg and a pulmonary capillary wedge pressure less than 15 mmHg by right heart catheterization define PAH. Increased pulmonary vascular resistance due to vasoconstriction characterizes pulmonary hypertension and remodelling of the vessel wall, reflected by intima thickening, media hypertrophy and endothelial cell dysfunction. These changes reflect the imbalance between local vasoconstrictors (endothelin 1) and vasodilators (prostacyclin and nitric oxide). The consequent increase in pulmonary vascular resistance leads to right cardiac insufficiency and death.

The estimated prevalence of PAH in SSc patients is about 10–12 %, with worst survival rates than idiopathic PAH or PAH associated with other connective tissue diseases. Mortality rate was until recently estimated around 50–55 % at 1 year [48], but clearly improved due to systematic screening and available therapeutic armamentarium.

Several methods have been developed to assess subclinical atherosclerosis. Increased carotid intima-media thickness (IMT) and impaired endothelial-dependent flow-mediated dilation (FMD) both correlate with traditional CV risk factors and predict vascular events in general population. In SSc, IMT is higher and FMD lower than in general population again suggesting an increased prevalence of subclinical atherosclerosis [44]. Also arterial stiffness is increased in the presence of traditional CV risk factors and is an independent predictor of CV events and mortality. In SSc, varying results were encountered in this index, some revealing elevated arterial stiffness and with correlation to soluble markers of endothelial activation. Coronary calcium score as detected by multidetector computed tomography measuring coronary artery calcification that occurs in atherosclerotic plaque has also been studied in SSc, but its increased prevalence has still an unknown relation to angiographic findings.

Traditional Cardiovascular Risk Factors

Traditional cardiovascular risk factors in SSc should always be addressed and controlled, although their contribution for CV risk does not fully account for the overall increased morbidity [49]. It is recognized that lipid profile including increased LDL, hyperhomocysteinaemia, folate and vitamin B12 deficiency are players in the complex endothelial injury present in these patients [39].

Nontraditional Biomarkers

Several pro-inflammatory mediators have been studied as active participants in vascular injury. The most known and widely available for measurement is C-reactive protein, although its predictive value for CV morbidity remains unknown. More recently, N-terminal pro-brain natriuretic peptide (NT-proBNP) levels demonstrated to have a good correlation to cardiac filling pressures and ventricular stress [50] and to be a predictor of cardiovascular events. NT-proBNP levels are raised in patients with cardiac failure and in patients with PAH, and as such, NT-proBNP arises as a very promising diagnostic and prognostic marker for ventricular dysfunction and pulmonary hypertension [51]. Though not available for assessment in daily clinical practice, several biomarkers, namely, IL-1, IL-6, macrophage migration inhibitory factor (MIF), monocyte chemoattractant protein 1 (MCP-1), endothelin 1 (ET-1), nitric oxide (NO), nitric oxide synthetase inhibitor asymmetric dimethylarginine (ADMA), soluble adhesion molecules (sICAM-1, sVCAM-1 and E-selectin), anti-endothelial cell antibodies (AECA) and vascular endothelial growth factor (VEGF), were independently associated with subclinical atherosclerosis in SSc patients [45, 47].

SSc Medication

SSc has still a paucity of truly disease-modifying antirheumatic drugs. Been a rare disease and until recently without consensus guidelines, it is difficult to assess the contribution of SSc medication to the CV risk. Corticosteroids are usually avoided, and immunosuppression, using different drugs, can be introduced depending on the type and severity of organ involvement. A recent study addressing CHD in SSc tried to elucidate about immunosuppression impact in CHD but failed to demonstrate decreased risks of acute myocardial infarction in patients taking penicillamine, systemic steroids, cyclophosphamide, azathioprine, methotrexate, or cyclosporine [52].

Calcium channel blockers and angiotensin-converting enzyme inhibitors play a role in the treatment of microvascular ischemia in systemic sclerosis patients and may have a beneficial, though not documented, effect on CV protection.

Primary Sjögren's Syndrome

Primary Sjögren's syndrome (pSS) is an immune-mediated disease characterized by chronic inflammation of the exocrine glands and the presence of autoantibodies anti-SSA/Ro and anti-SSB/La.

There are no conclusive data on CV mortality, and information on the actual CV risk in pSS is limited. However, a recently presented population-based study from British Columbia, Canada, found a significantly increased risk of MI, particularly in the first year following diagnosis, and a trend towards an increased risk for stoke [11].

Signs of premature subclinical atherosclerosis have also been shown in pSS patients, including enhanced carotid and femoral IMT, arterial stiffness and more frequent abnormal ankle-brachial index. Greater IMT is associated with the presence of anti-SSA antibodies and leukopenia/lymphopenia, suggesting that immune dysregulation might promote atherosclerosis in pSS [53]. Curiously, the prevalence of atherosclerotic plaques in pSS and controls is similar.

Much remains to be learned about traditional and nontraditional CV risk factors in this disease. Some research groups demonstrated a higher prevalence of diabetes and hypertriglyceridaemia, predominantly in patients receiving corticosteroids. Hypertension was also found to be 2 times more prevalent in pSS than in controls. Low levels of total and HDL cholesterol were reported in pSS, and abnormal lipid profile was substantially more frequent in patients with anti-SSA/SSB antibodies, but the contribution of these alterations to subclinical atherosclerosis appears to be marginal. Surrogate markers of endothelial dysfunction, such as the number of endothelial progenitor cells, endothelial microparticles and ADMA levels, are altered in pSS patients [19].

Although a bulk of evidence suggests that CV risk is higher among pSS patients, results must be interpreted with caution since the majority of studies include only few patients and need to be replicated in larger cohorts.

Systemic Vasculitis

Systemic vasculitis is by definition characterized by inflammation of the blood vessel wall that causes thickening, narrowing or weakening of the vessel wall. The Chapel Hill Consensus conference classifies vasculitis according to vessel size involvement into large-, medium- and small-vessel vasculitis, although overlap between most entities is recognized. The clinical manifestations and complications result from restriction of blood flow and depend on the type, size and localization of the affected vessels. As expected, vasculitis per se can cause CV complications such as stroke, MI, arterial aneurisms or dissection. Moreover, hypertension is common in vasculitis affecting the renal arteries. The question whether atherogenesis is more frequent in this group of systemic inflammatory disorders remains controversial.

Cardiovascular complications such as stroke, aortic aneurisms and dissection are classically related to large-vessel vasculitis as giant cell arteritis (GCA), but in a population-based incidence cohort, the overall risk of acute coronary syndromes in patients diagnosed with GCA between 1950 and 2009 was not increased compared to controls from the same population with similar age, sex and calendar year [12]. Although epidemiological studies demonstrated increased risk of stroke, in particular in the vertebra-basilar territory, no increase in the overall mortality seems to be associated with GCA [9]. Moreover, a small case-control study didn't show significant differences in IMT between patients with GCA and controls [54].

A review about another large-vessel vasculitis – Takayasu arteritis (TA) – depicted accelerated atherosclerosis, higher IMT, greater arterial stiffness and higher prevalence of carotid plaques compared to matched controls in vasculitis-affected arteries. TA patients have 10–20 % risk of stroke and 10–30 % risk of coronary artery disease.

Kawasaki disease is known for its cardiovascular complications that include coronary artery aneurisms, but is still controversial if associated with accelerated atherosclerosis.

ANCA-associated vasculitis during active phase may have accelerated atherosclerosis that ameliorates with disease control. Nevertheless, vessel damage may subside and aggravate with disease reactivations. Therefore, theses patients have increased late mortality due to cardiovascular disease and a two- to fourfold increase in CHD, probably related to disease burden.

Traditional Cardiovascular Risk Factors

Lipid profile may be altered in systemic vasculitis especially regarding HDL subsets and pro-inflammatory LDL but without clear clinical relation to CV events. Due to the fact that these patients are treated with high doses of corticosteroids, it is very difficult to separate what is the effect of disease from the effect of treatment in atherogenesis.

Nontraditional Biomarkers

Besides LDL particles, other oxidized products and modified phospholipids can promote inflammatory responses through endothelial and macrophage activation, and the oxidized proteins may become immunogenic.

Vasculitis Medication

The information regarding the effect of vasculitis medication on atherosclerosis is scarce. In theory, immunosuppressants could decrease CV risk by suppressing systemic inflammation as well as cardiac and vascular inflammation, and in fact it was demonstrated that endothelial dysfunction normalizes with corticosteroid therapy in GCA.

Low-dose aspirin has been recommended in large-vessel vasculitis in an attempt to reduce ischemic complications, without strong evidence supporting its benefits. Nonsteroidal anti-inflammatory drugs (NSAIDs) also may contribute to the reduction of atherosclerotic lesion formation and destabilization.

Statins should be considered depending on the side effect risk due to its positive effect on endothelial progenitor cells and inhibition of inflammation (Table 6.2).

Table 6.2 Summary of novel cardiovascular biomarkers identified in rheumatic diseases and their association with vascular disease

	SLE	RA	pSS	SSc	Vasculitis
CRP	+/–	+	+	+	–
piHDL	+	+	N/A	N/A	N/A
E-selectin	+	+	N/A	N/A	N/A
sICAM-1	+	+	N/A	+	N/A
VCAM	+/–	+	N/A	N/A	–
EPC	+	+	+	+	+
TM	+	+	N/A	+	–
TF	+	+	N/A	N/A	N/A
vWF	+	+	N/A	N/A	–
PAI-1	N/A	+	N/A	+	N/A
IL-1	+/–	+	+	N/A	N/A
IL-6	+	+	+	+	N/A
MIF	+	+	+	N/A	N/A
MCP-1	+	+	+	N/A	N/A
ADMA	+	+	+	+	N/A
NT-proBNP	–	+	+	+	N/A

SLE systemic lupus erythematosus, *RA* rheumatoid arthritis, *SSc* systemic sclerosis, *pSS* primary Sjögren's syndrome, *CRP* C-reactive protein, *IL* interleukin, *TM* thrombomodulin, *TF* tissue factor, *EPC* endothelial progenitor cells, *vWF* von Willebrand's factor, *PAI* plasminogen activator inhibitor, *piHDL* pro-inflammatory HDL, *ADMA* asymmetric dimethylarginine, *NT-proBNP* N-terminal pro-brain natriuretic peptide, *MCP* monocyte chemoattractant protein, *sICAM* soluble intercellular adhesion molecule, *VCAM* vascular cell adhesion molecule, *MIF* macrophage migration inhibitory factor

+ positive association; +/– conflicting results; – no association; N/A no information available

Conclusion

Cardiovascular burden is substantially increased in several immune-mediated rheumatic diseases. Physicians must be aware of this excessive risk and the need for its systematic evaluation and tight control.

Traditional CV risk factors are highly prevalent in systemic rheumatic diseases and may be worsened by disease activity or by the use of some antirheumatic medications. Nevertheless, the disproportionate CV risk cannot be totally explained by the presence of CV risk factors, and tools for risk stratification used in the general population do not perform well in systemic inflammatory disorders.

Many studies identified biomarkers of endothelial activation, oxidative stress, inflammatory mediators and haemostatic factors associated with atherosclerosis in rheumatic diseases, but while numerous surrogate markers of atherosclerosis have been described in RA, SLE, pSS, SSc and systemic vasculitis, their usefulness in clinical practice remains uncertain. Currently, the best strategy for the management of CV risk associated with rheumatic diseases is the strict control of inflammatory disease activity and the regular screening and treatment of associated CV risk factors.

References

1. Bernatsky S, Boivin J-F, Joseph L, Manzi S, Ginzler E, Gladman DD, et al. Mortality in systemic lupus erythematosus. Arthritis Rheum [Internet]. 2006;54(8):2550–7. Available from: http://www.ncbi.nlm.nih.gov/pubmed/16868977. Cited 14 Sept 2014.
2. Aviña-Zubieta JA, Choi HK, Sadatsafavi M, Etminan M, Esdaile JM, Lacaille D. Risk of cardiovascular mortality in patients with rheumatoid arthritis: a meta-analysis of observational studies. Arthritis Rheum [Internet]. 2008;59(12):1690–7. Available from: http://www.ncbi.nlm.nih.gov/pubmed/19035419. Cited 18 Oct 2014.
3. Gonzalez A, Maradit Kremers H, Crowson CS, Nicola PJ, Davis JM, Therneau TM, et al. The widening mortality gap between rheumatoid arthritis patients and the general population. Arthritis Rheum [Internet]. 2007;56(11):3583–7. Available from: http://www.ncbi.nlm.nih.gov/pubmed/17968923. Cited 18 Oct 2014.
4. Manzi S, Meilahn EN, Rairie JE, Conte CG, Medsger TA, Jansen-McWilliams L, et al. Age-specific incidence rates of myocardial infarction and angina in women with systemic lupus erythematosus: comparison with the Framingham Study. Am J Epidemiol [Internet]. 1997;145(5):408–15. Available from: http://aje.oxfordjournals.org/cgi/doi/10.1093/oxfordjournals.aje.a009122.
5. Schoenfeld SR, Kasturi S, Costenbader KH. The epidemiology of atherosclerotic cardiovascular disease among patients with SLE: a systematic review. Semin Arthritis Rheum [Internet]. Elsevier. 2013;43(1):77–95. Available from: http://www.ncbi.nlm.nih.gov/pubmed/23422269. Cited 18 Oct 2014.
6. Avina-Zubieta JA, Thomas J, Sadatsafavi M, Lehman AJ, Lacaille D. Risk of incident cardiovascular events in patients with rheumatoid arthritis: a meta-analysis of observational studies. Ann Rheum Dis [Internet]. 2012;71:1524–9. Available from: http://www.ncbi.nlm.nih.gov/pubmed/22425941.
7. Ungprasert P, Charoenpong P, Ratanasrimetha P, Thongprayoon C, Cheungpasitporn W, Suksaranjit P. Risk of coronary artery disease in patients with systemic sclerosis: A systematic review and meta-analysis. Clin Rheumatol [Internet]. Springer-Verlag London Ltd; 2014;33(8):1099–104. Available from: http://www.ncbi.nlm.nih.gov/pubmed/24859783. Cited 18 Oct 2014.
8. Chiang C-H, Liu C-J, Huang C-C, Chan W-L, Huang P-H, Chen T-J, et al. Systemic sclerosis and risk of ischaemic stroke: a nationwide cohort study. Rheumatology (Oxford) [Internet]. 2013;52:161–5. Available from: http://www.ncbi.nlm.nih.gov/pubmed/23238980.
9. Cohen Tervaert JW. Cardiovascular disease due to accelerated atherosclerosis in systemic vasculitides. Best Pract Res Clin Rheumatol. 2013;27:33–44.
10. Faurschou M, Mellemkjaer L, Sorensen IJ, Thomsen BS, Dreyer L, Baslund B. Increased morbidity from ischemic heart disease in patients with Wegener's granulomatosis. Arthritis Rheum. 2009;60:1187–92.
11. Yurkovich M, Sayre EC, Shojania K, Avina-Zubieta JA. The risk of myocardial infarction and cerebrovascular accident in patients with Sjogren's syndrome: a general population-based cohort study. Ann Rheum Dis [Internet]. 2014;73(Suppl 2):142–143. Available from: 10.1136/annrheumdis-2014-eular.3108.
12. Udayakumar PD, Chandran AK, Crowson CS, Warrington KJ, Matteson EL. Cardiovascular risk and acute coronary syndrome in giant cell arteritis: a population based retrospective

cohort study. Arthritis Care Res (Hoboken) [Internet]. 2015;67(3):396–02. Available from: http://dx.doi.org/10.1002/acr.22416.
13. Symmons DPM, Gabriel SE. Epidemiology of CVD in rheumatic disease, with a focus on RA and SLE. Nat Rev Rheumatol [Internet]. Nature Publishing Group. 2011;7(7):399–408. Available from: http://www.ncbi.nlm.nih.gov/pubmed/21629241. Cited 18 Oct 2014.
14. Ibañez D, Gladman DD, Urowitz MB. Adjusted mean systemic lupus erythematosus disease activity index-2K is a predictor of outcome in SLE. J Rheumatol. 2005;32(5):824–7.
15. Steiman AJ, Gladman DD, Ibañez D, Urowitz MB. Outcomes in patients with systemic lupus erythematosus with and without a prolonged serologically active clinically quiescent period. Arthritis Care Res. 2012;64:511–8.
16. Del Rincón I, Polak JF, O'Leary DH, Battafarano DF, Erikson JM, Restrepo JF, et al. Systemic inflammation and cardiovascular risk factors predict rapid progression of atherosclerosis in rheumatoid arthritis. Ann Rheum Dis [Internet]. 2014. Available from: http://ard.bmj.com/content/early/2014/05/20/annrheumdis-2013-205058.abstract.
17. Santos MJ, Carmona-Fernandes D, Canhão H, Canas da Silva J, Fonseca JE, Gil V. Early vascular alterations in SLE and RA patients – a step towards understanding the associated cardiovascular risk. PLoS One [Internet]. 2012;7(9):e44668. Available from: http://www.pubmedcentral.nih.gov/articlerender.fcgi?artid=3433444&tool=pmcentrez&rendertype=abstract. Cited 18 Oct 2014.
18. Rodríguez-Carrio J, Prado C, de Paz B, López P, Gómez J, Alperi-López M, et al. Circulating endothelial cells and their progenitors in systemic lupus erythematosus and early rheumatoid arthritis patients. Rheumatology (Oxford) [Internet]. 2012;51:1775–84. Available from: http://www.ncbi.nlm.nih.gov/pubmed/22753774.
19. Bartoloni E, Alunno A, Bistoni O, Caterbi S, Luccioli F, Santoboni G, et al. Characterization of circulating endothelial microparticles and endothelial progenitor cells in primary Sjögren's syndrome: new markers of chronic endothelial damage? Rheumatol [Internet]. 2014. Available from: http://rheumatology.oxfordjournals.org/content/early/2014/09/04/rheumatology.keu320.abstract.
20. Koenig W, Ernst E. The possible role of hemorheology in atherothrombogenesis. Atherosclerosis. 1992;94:93–107.
21. Santos MJ, Pedro LM, Canhão H, Fernandes E, Fernandes J, Canas da Silva J, Fonseca JE, et al. Hemorheological parameters are related to subclinical atherosclerosis in systemic lupus erythematosus and rheumatoid arthritis patients. Atherosclerosis [Internet]. 2011;219(2):821–6. Available from: http://www.ncbi.nlm.nih.gov/pubmed/21906736. Cited 18 Oct 2014.
22. Westphal JR, Boerbooms AM, Schalwijk CJ, Kwast H, De Weijert M, Jacobs C, et al. Anti-endothelial cell antibodies in sera of patients with autoimmune diseases: comparison between ELISA and FACS analysis. Clin Exp Immunol. 1994;96:444–9.
23. Fesmire J, Wolfson-Reichlin M, Reichlin M. Effects of autoimmune antibodies anti-lipoprotein lipase, anti-low density lipoprotein, and anti-oxidized low density lipoprotein on lipid metabolism and atherosclerosis in systemic lupus erythematosus. Rev Bras Reumatol. 2010;50:545–51.
24. Batuca JR, Ames PRJ, Isenberg DA, Delgado Alves J. Antibodies toward high-density lipoprotein components inhibit paraoxonase activity in patients with systemic lupus erythematosus. Ann N Y Acad Sci. 2007;1108:137–46.
25. Su J, Frostegård AG, Hua X, Gustafsson T, Jogestrand T, Hafström I, et al. Low levels of antibodies against oxidized but not nonoxidized cardiolipin and phosphatidylserine are associated with atherosclerotic plaques in systemic lupus erythematosus. J Rheumatol. 2013;40:1856–64.
26. Majka DS, Liu K, Pope RM, Karlson EW, Vu T-HT, Teodorescu M, et al. Antiphospholipid antibodies and sub-clinical atherosclerosis in the Coronary Artery Risk Development in Young Adults (CARDIA) cohort. Inflamm Res [Internet]. 2013;62:919–27. Available from: http://www.ncbi.nlm.nih.gov/pubmed/23959159.

27. Westlake SL, Colebatch AN, Baird J, Kiely P, Quinn M, Choy E, et al. The effect of methotrexate on cardiovascular disease in patients with rheumatoid arthritis: a systematic literature review. Rheumatology (Oxford) [Internet]. 2010;49(2):295–307. Available from: http://www.ncbi.nlm.nih.gov/pubmed/19946022. Cited 15 Oct 2014.
28. Micha R, Imamura F, Wyler Von Ballmoos M, Solomon DH, Hernán MA, Ridker PM, et al. Systematic review and meta-analysis of methotrexate use and risk of cardiovascular disease. Am J Cardiol. 2011;108:1362–70.
29. Hjeltnes G, Hollan I, Førre Ø, Wiik A, Lyberg T, Mikkelsen K, et al. Endothelial function improves within 6 weeks of treatment with methotrexate or methotrexate in combination with a TNF-α inhibitor in rheumatoid arthritis patients. Scand J Rheumatol [Internet]. Informa Healthcare; 2012;41(3):240–2. Available from: http://dx.doi.org/10.3109/03009742.2012.656698.
30. Tam LS, Kitas GD, Gonźlez-gay MA. Can suppression of inflammation by anti-TNF prevent progression of subclinical atherosclerosis in inflammatory arthritis? Rheumatology (Oxford). 2014;53:1108–19.
31. Barnabe C, Martin B-J, Ghali WA. Systematic review and meta-analysis: anti-tumor necrosis factor α therapy and cardiovascular events in rheumatoid arthritis. Arthritis Care Res (Hoboken) [Internet]. 2011;63(4):522–9. Available from: http://www.ncbi.nlm.nih.gov/pubmed/20957658. Cited 16 Oct 2014.
32. Roman MJ, Moeller E, Davis A, Paget SA, Crow MK, Lockshin MD, et al. Preclinical carotid atherosclerosis in patients with rheumatoid arthritis. Ann Intern Med. 2006;144(4):249–56.
33. Kao AH, Wasko MCM, Krishnaswami S, Wagner J, Edmundowicz D, Shaw P, et al. C-reactive protein and coronary artery calcium in asymptomatic women with systemic lupus erythematosus or rheumatoid arthritis. Am J Cardiol. 2008;102:755–60.
34. Kerekes G, Szekanecz Z, Dér H, Sándor Z, Lakos G, Muszbek L, et al. Endothelial dysfunction and atherosclerosis in rheumatoid arthritis: a multiparametric analysis using imaging techniques and laboratory markers of inflammation and autoimmunity. J Rheumatol. 2008;35:398–406.
35. Manzi S, Meilahn EN, Rairie JE, Conte CG, Medsger T a., Jansen-McWilliams L, et al. Age-specific Incidence Rates of Myocardial Infarction and Angina in Women with Systemic Lupus Erythematosus: Comparison with the Framingham Study. Am J Epidemiol [Internet]. 1997;145(5):408–15. Available from: http://aje.oxfordjournals.org/cgi/doi/10.1093/oxfordjournals.aje.a009122
36. Hachulla E, Coghlan JG. A new era in the management of pulmonary arterial hypertension related to scleroderma: endothelin receptor antagonism. Ann Rheum Dis. 2004;63:1009–14.
37. Tamby MC, Chanseaud Y, Guillevin L, Mouthon L. New insights into the pathogenesis of systemic sclerosis. Autoimmun Rev. 2003;2:152–7.
38. Jara LJ, Medina G, Vera-Lastra O, Amigo MC. Accelerated atherosclerosis, immune response and autoimmune rheumatic diseases. Autoimmun Rev. 2006;5:195–201.
39. Szekanecz Z, Koch AE. Vascular involvement in rheumatic diseases: "vascular rheumatology". Arthritis Res Ther [Internet]. 2008;10(5):224. Available from: http://www.pubmedcentral.nih.gov/articlerender.fcgi?artid=2592799&tool=pmcentrez&rendertype=abstract. Cited 18 Oct 2014.
40. Tyndall AJ, Bannert B, Vonk M, Airò P, Cozzi F, Carreira PE, et al. Causes and risk factors for death in systemic sclerosis: a study from the EULAR Scleroderma Trials and Research (EUSTAR) database. Ann Rheum Dis. 2010;69:1809–15.
41. Dave AJ, Fiorentino D, Lingala B, Krishnan E, Chung L. Atherosclerotic cardiovascular disease in hospitalized patients with systemic sclerosis: higher mortality than patients with lupus and rheumatoid arthritis. Arthritis Care Res (Hoboken) [Internet]. 2014;66:323–7. Available from: http://www.ncbi.nlm.nih.gov/pubmed/24022876.
42. Allanore Y, Meune C. Primary myocardial involvement in systemic sclerosis: evidence for a microvascular origin. Clin Exp Rheumatol. 2010;28(5 Suppl 62):S48–53.

43. Man A, Zhu Y, Zhang Y, Dubreuil M, Rho YH, Peloquin C, et al. The risk of cardiovascular disease in systemic sclerosis: a population-based cohort study. Ann Rheum Dis [Internet]. 2013;72:1188–93. Available from: http://www.ncbi.nlm.nih.gov/pubmed/22904260.
44. Ngian G-S, Sahhar J, Proudman SM, Stevens W, Wicks IP, Van Doornum S. Prevalence of coronary heart disease and cardiovascular risk factors in a national cross-sectional cohort study of systemic sclerosis. Ann Rheum Dis [Internet]. 2012;71:1980–3. Available from: http://www.ncbi.nlm.nih.gov/pubmed/22532628.
45. Ngian G-S, Sahhar J, Wicks IP, Van Doornum S. Cardiovascular disease in systemic sclerosis – an emerging association? Arthritis Res Ther [Internet]. 2011;13:237. Available from: http://www.pubmedcentral.nih.gov/articlerender.fcgi?artid=3239376&tool=pmcentrez&rendertype=abstract.
46. Ho M, Veale D, Eastmond C, Nuki G, Belch J. Macrovascular disease and systemic sclerosis. Ann Rheum Dis. 2000;59:39–43.
47. Schiopu E, Au KM, Mcmahon MA, Kaplan MJ, Divekar A, Singh RR, et al. Prevalence of subclinical atherosclerosis is increased in systemic sclerosis and is associated with serum proteins: a cross-sectional, controlled study of carotid ultrasound. Rheumatology (Oxford). 2014;53:704–13.
48. Hachulla E, Carpentier P, Gressin V, Diot E, Allanore Y, Sibilia J, et al. Risk factors for death and the 3-year survival of patients with systemic sclerosis: the French ItinerAIR-Sclerodermie study. Rheumatology. 2009;48:304–8.
49. Shoenfeld Y, Gerli R, Doria A, Matsuura E, Cerinic MM, Ronda N, et al. Accelerated atherosclerosis in autoimmune rheumatic diseases. Circulation [Internet]. 2005;112(21):3337–47. Available from: http://www.ncbi.nlm.nih.gov/pubmed/16301360. Cited 20 Sept 2014.
50. Groenning BA, Raymond I, Hildebrandt PR, Nilsson JC, Baumann M, Pedersen F. Diagnostic and prognostic evaluation of left ventricular systolic heart failure by plasma N-terminal pro-brain natriuretic peptide concentrations in a large sample of the general population. Heart. 2004;90:297–303.
51. Allanore Y, Borderie D, Meune C, Cabanes L, Weber S, Ekindjian OG, et al. N-terminal pro-brain natriuretic peptide as a diagnostic marker of early pulmonary artery hypertension in patients with systemic sclerosis and effects of calcium-channel blockers. Arthritis Rheum. 2003;48:3503–8.
52. Chu S-Y, Chen Y-J, Liu C-J, Tseng W-C, Lin M-W, Hwang C-Y, et al. Increased risk of acute myocardial infarction in systemic sclerosis: a nationwide population-based study. Am J Med [Internet]. Elsevier; 2014;126(11):982–8. Available from: http://www.amjmed.com/article/S0002-9343(13)00593-7/abstract.
53. Vaudo G, Bocci EB, Shoenfeld Y, Schillaci G, Wu R, Del Papa N, et al. Precocious intima-media thickening in patients with primary Sjögren's syndrome. Arthritis Rheum. 2005;52:3890–7.
54. Gonzalez-Juanatey C, Lopez-Diaz MJ, Martin J, Llorca J, Gonzalez-Gay MA. Atherosclerosis in patients with biopsy-proven giant cell arteritis. Arthritis Rheum. 2007;57:1481–6.

Chapter 7
Cardiometabolic Risk, Inflammation, and Neurodegenerative Disorders

Filipe Palavra, Ethel Ciampi Díaz, and Armando Sena

Abstract Inflammation has been recognized as an important character in the underlying mechanisms leading to the development of various types of neurodegenerative disorders. In this sense, both inflammation of the nervous system itself and systemic inflammation act in the complex pathophysiology of these neurological diseases. The nervous system does not play a passive role in the complexity of these mechanisms and can itself be responsible for perpetuating pro-inflammatory stimuli – it is today recognized the important role that specific brain areas play in the so-called metabolic inflammation. This dialectical relationship will be the focus of this chapter.

Keywords Inflammation • Inflammation mediators • Metabolic syndrome • Neurodegenerative diseases • Alzheimer's disease • Multiple sclerosis

In recent years, the advancement of scientific knowledge has assigned a key role to inflammation in the mechanisms leading to the development of neurodegenerative diseases. It is now known that, in these processes, it is not only inflammation restricted to the central nervous system (CNS) that is involved, but there is actually a two-way relationship between the CNS and systemic inflammatory environment, so that the activity of each of them mutually influences.

That will be the central concept of this chapter, which is divided into two parts. At first, we will focus our attention on the mechanisms of brain inflammation

F. Palavra, M.D. (✉)
Laboratory of Pharmacology and Experimental Therapeutics, Institute for Biomedical Imaging and Life Sciences (IBILI) and CNC.IBILI Research Unit, Faculty of Medicine, Sub-Unit 1, Pólo 3, Coimbra University, Azinhaga de Santa Comba – Celas, 3000-548 Coimbra, Portugal
e-mail: filipepalavra@uc.pt

E.C. Díaz, M.D.
Department of Neurology, Hospital Clinico
Pontificia Universidad Catolica de Chile, Santiago, Chile

A. Sena, M.D., Ph.D.
Interdisciplinary Centre of Research Egas Moniz, CiiEM, Caparica, Portugal

© Springer International Publishing Switzerland 2015
F. Palavra et al. (eds.), *Biomarkers of Cardiometabolic Risk, Inflammation and Disease*, DOI 10.1007/978-3-319-16018-4_7

induced by overnutrition, a topic that, over the last decade, has allowed a fruitful advancement of knowledge in the field of metabolic syndrome and its related disorders. A more mechanistic view will be presented, using data mainly coming from research of more fundamental characteristics, as this is in fact an area of very recent development and that, in the future, will certainly contribute to a better understanding of the highly complex and clinically heterogeneous metabolic disorders. In the second part of the chapter, we will focus on aspects of clinical nature, related to some diseases that have, in their pathophysiology, neurodegenerative features. In fact, at older ages or still in youth, inflammation and cardiometabolic risk may influence the progression of such diseases and, thus, limit the quality of life of patients and the prognosis itself, at short, medium, or long term.

It is important, therefore, to reflect on these aspects. Also in the case of neurodegenerative diseases, the tight control of cardiometabolic risk factors may have significant clinical impact. A better understanding of the intricate relationship between inflammation, cardiometabolic risk, and neurodegeneration can help to optimize the clinical management of such diseases and thereby improve the quality of life of our patients, the core of all our concerns as medical doctors.

Brain Dysfunction: Cause or Consequence of Overnutrition-Induced Diseases?

The history of the human species has always been characterized by a significant expenditure of effort in gathering enough food for survival. However, the high energy consumption required to keep all the energy-producing mechanisms functioning was dramatically changed by modern industrialization, becoming relatively easy for any individual, after that, to quickly obtain calorie-abundant food. This deep change in the process of food demand and in diet itself introduced some medical problems in modern societies, which have started to face true epidemics of overnutrition-related diseases such as obesity, type 2 diabetes *mellitus* (T2D), and cardiovascular diseases (CVD) [1–3]. The social and economic model of human feeding has changed so much that it is now virtually impossible to think on returning to the hunter-gatherers' way of life, but the consequences of the diseases mentioned above for public health have been so devastating that, at least in theory, it would not be totally inappropriate to think in going back a few decades.

From the pathophysiological perspective, outbursts of those diseases are frequently preceded by a complex derangement of a constellation of metabolic parameters including obesity, insulin resistance leading to glucose tolerance impairment, dyslipidemia, and arterial hypertension, defining, as a whole, the so-called metabolic syndrome (MetS) [4]. Logically, any early therapeutic and preventive strategy demonstrating to be effective against MetS could have a tremendous impact on public health, controlling the myriad of dangerous outcomes of T2D and CVD. Nevertheless, the understanding of the root mechanisms of all these disorders is still insufficient to allow us to treat our patients with an extremely effective and potent miraculous drug. But, in the last decade, studies coming from the fields of endocrinology and immunology started to change this figure, and some developments have been made, principally related to the recognition that overnutrition is an environmental factor targeted by the innate immune system, which triggers an atypical form of inflammation (the so-called metabolic inflammation) that is responsible for some degree of metabolic dysfunctions at subcellular, cellular, organ, and systemic levels [5]. Under nutritional excess, such kind of inflammation is mainly driving the generation of various intracellular stresses (mitochondrial oxidative stress, endoplasmic reticulum stress, and autophagy defect) and those abnormalities have been established to occur not only at a peripheral level but also in the CNS. In fact, one of the first reports of an association existing between obesity and brain structural and biochemical alterations was published by Sena et al., in the early 1980s [6]: leptin-deficient mice developed systemic metabolic disturbances suggestive of primary hypothalamic dysfunction. Hypothalamus is recognized as a true metabolic center, governing various activities of the body, such as temperature, blood pressure, and appetite control. Its role in carbohydrate and lipid metabolism, controlling the energy consumption of the body, has received much attention in recent years, making the hypothalamus an extremely attractive target for drug development in MetS [7].

It is very common to find personal trainers who, in weight loss programs, often refer to "be all inside the head" of their pupils. Research in this area has clearly demonstrated that, at least in part, this statement is not devoid of truth. In the following sections, recent achievements will be discussed, clarifying the role of inflammation and brain stress (particularly at a hypothalamic level) in MetS.

The Hypothalamus Is a Key Region for Energy Balance Regulation

The hypothalamus is a brain structure located below the thalamus (as the name implies), comprising the major portion of the ventral diencephalon. Its anatomical organization is defined by a set of distinct nuclei, which correspond to neuronal clusters responsible for specific homeostatic functions, principally related to the regulation of endocrine axes and energy balance. Neurons contained in these nuclei contribute to form interconnected circuits via axonal projections and respond to changes in energy status by altering the production of specific neurotransmitters and neuromodulators and thus changing energy intake and expenditure accordingly [8].

The arcuate nucleus (ARC) is considered to be the principal responsible for food intake control. It contains two different populations of neurons receiving feeding signals from the periphery: one set of neurons produces the orexigenic (feeding-promoting) neuropeptides agouti-related protein (AgRP) and neuropeptide Y (NPY), and the second group of neurons produces the anorexigenic (feeding inhibitors) products of proopiomelanocortin (POMC), the precursor of alpha-melanocyte stimulating hormone (α-MSH) and the cocaine and amphetamine-regulated transcript (CART). The orexigenic neurons project their axons mainly to other hypothalamic nuclei, such as the paraventricular nucleus (PVH), but the anorexigenic ones have a broader distribution, making connections with the dorsomedial nucleus (DMH), the lateral hypothalamic area (LHA), the perifornical area, the PVH, and the other areas of the CNS. The ARC is also connected with the ventromedial hypothalamus (VMH), whose neurons project their axons to the DMH, the LHA, and the ARC itself and to the brainstem, namely, to the nucleus of the solitary tract.

These hypothalamic neurons are able to change their activity and the synthesis of neuropeptides in response to different peripheral signals, such as glucose, lipids, amino acids, and hormones (like insulin, leptin, ghrelin, adiponectin, resistin, and glucagon-like peptide-1). When the supply of energy to the body exceeds its real needs, the synthesis of orexigenic neuropeptides (AgRP and NPY) decreases. On the other hand, when the energy input is insufficient and expenditure surpasses feeding, the production of anorexigenic neuropeptides diminishes and the tone is placed on the orexigenic ones [8, 9].

Brain/Hypothalamic Stress and Metabolic Syndrome

There are fundamentally three types of mechanisms for inducing stress in brain cells that may have implications in the relationship of the brain itself (particularly of the hypothalamic neurons) with the MetS: oxidative stress, endoplasmic reticulum stress, and autophagy defect.

The brain uses a large amount of oxygen and ATP to ensure its normal activity and functions and, therefore, is highly susceptible to oxidative stress, mainly mediated by reactive oxygen species (ROS). ROS refer to a class of radical or non-radical oxygen-containing molecules that have high oxidative reactivity with carbon-containing substances like lipids, proteins, and nucleic acids. There are many possible sources of ROS in cells, but the mitochondria, which generates energy in the form of ATP using oxygen, is one of the most relevant ROS-generating cellular organelles (in fact, the largest amount of intracellular ROS comes directly from the leakage of mitochondrial electron transport chain). Other sources of ROS are enzymes involved in specific metabolic processes, such as nicotinamide adenine dinucleotide phosphate (NADPH) oxidase, cyclooxygenases, lipoxygenases, xanthine oxidase, and enzymes related to the cytochrome p450 complex [10]. Considering that the production of ROS is physiologically unavoidable, cells are equipped with a battery of antioxidant enzymes that keep their levels controlled and within a range not considered a threat to cellular homeostasis (such kind of enzymes are, e.g., superoxide dismutases, catalases, and aldehyde dehydrogenases). It is worth to say that, more recently, the evil profile of ROS has been changing, since the discovery that physiological levels of intracellular ROS can be normally involved in some functions, such as kinase proteins activation, ion transport across membranes, regulation of gene expression, and generation of intracellular calcium waves [11].

However, when ROS homeostasis is disturbed (due to several environmental or pathological factors), they are easily accumulated in the mitochondria and in the cytoplasm and they start to induce oxidative stress in the cell, causing dysfunction and disease. Indeed, the development of some neurodegenerative diseases is believed to be fostered by oxidative stress, suggesting that the CNS is highly susceptible to this phenomenon [12]. The role of brain (and particularly hypothalamic) oxidative stress in the pathogenesis of MetS is not yet sufficiently and deeply known to assume a causal relationship, but there is some evidence published in favor of this hypothesis. For example, it was possible to induce the activity of NADPH oxidase in rat brains by dietary obesity [13]. It was also shown that mitochondrial dysfunction in hypothalamic POMC neurons compromises the mechanisms of central glucose homeostasis [14] and that the deletion of peroxisome proliferator-activated receptor coactivator 1α (PGC-1α) also generates mitochondrial dysfunction and a disruption of central regulation of energy balance [15]. The role of brain oxidative stress in the development of MetS is, therefore, an extremely attractive target for future research and, maybe, for the development of innovative therapeutic strategies.

Apart from oxidative stress, the dysfunction of other cellular organelle – the endoplasmic reticulum – may also contribute to the disruption of neuronal machinery in MetS. The endoplasmic reticulum is responsible for protein synthesis, maturation, and transport to secretory pathways in the cell. Under physiological conditions, this organelle uses its unfolded protein response (UPR) tool to perfectly adapt protein synthesis, folding, and secretion to cellular needs. However, when cellular metabolic changes occur, producing some instability in proteostasis, the endoplasmic reticulum increases its activity and the UPR may not be sufficient to neutralize this metabolism-induced stress. This unresolved endoplasmic reticulum stress may be sufficient to induce cell apoptosis, which may be related with the origin of some neurodegenerative diseases, diabetic islet cell death, and stroke, for example [16]. Endoplasmic reticulum stress may also contribute to the activation of cellular inflammatory pathways and to the accumulation of ROS, inducing also damage by oxidative stress (that can be synergistically responsible for the development of further metabolic derangements). This connection has been associated to obesity, insulin resistance, T2D, CVD, neurodegenerative disorders, and cancer [17].

Considering that, in recent years, the role of the brain in metabolic diseases has become a focus of scientific interest, the contribution of endoplasmic reticulum stress, particularly in the hypothalamus, has been progressively studied and characterized. In fact, some authors have causally linked brain endoplasmic reticulum stress under conditions of overnutrition and related inflammatory insults to the development of MetS, obesity, leptin and insulin resistance, dysfunction of the pancreatic β cell, and arterial hypertension [18–20]. These findings raised the possibility that endoplasmic reticulum stress could turn out to be also considered as a new therapeutic target in MetS.

The third mechanism that can be implicated in brain neuronal stress under metabolically demanding conditions is autophagy defect. Autophagy is a degradation pathway depending on lysosomal activity that plays a crucial role in maintaining homeostasis and promoting cell survival, differentiation, and growth [21], by cleaning up defective proteins or dysfunctional organelles. These functions are performed by three degradative systems – ubiquitin-proteasome system (UPS), chaperone-mediated autophagy (CMA), and macroautophagy. UPS is primarily responsible for degrading specific short-lived proteins, CMA only targets proteins containing particular peptide motifs, and macroautophagy has the capacity of eliminating long-lived cytosolic proteins and whole organelles [22]. Under normal circumstances, autophagy occurs at a basal level only to support cell growth and differentiation. However, if an environmental stress affects the cell (such as hypoxia), autophagic machinery is strongly induced to breakdown macromolecules into reusable fatty acids and amino acids, for survival. Thus, loss of autophagy control may become lethal to the cell [23].

Several pathologic conditions have been connected with tissue-specific impairment of autophagy: neurodegenerative diseases, heart diseases, cancer, and infection [24, 25]. Nevertheless, the role of brain autophagy defect in MetS is still scarcely studied although at least in theory would not be difficult to imagine a construct where autophagy defect could play a critical role in neuronal damage and such a construct could be based in several findings. In the first place, autophagy defect was already demonstrated to be implicated in cellular metabolic dysfunctions related with T2D and lipid disorder pathophysiology (that was observed in the liver, skeletal muscle, and pancreatic β cells) [26–28]. Second, a number of neurodegenerative diseases have been linked to a defective autophagic process in their pathophysiology, indicating the relevance of such cellular mechanisms for neuronal survival (examples are coming from the study of Alzheimer's, Parkinson's, and Huntington's diseases and transmissible spongiform encephalopathies) [29]. In fact, hypothalamic autophagy defect has already been linked to the development of obesity and insulin resistance, showing that a normal autophagic function is required for a correct energy homeostasis and a proper metabolic control [30]. Probably, the inducers of such a defect on the machinery guiding the autophagic processes are a prolonged exposition to oxidative stress (leading to intracellular accumulation of damaged mitochondria) and to endoplasmic reticulum stress (causing an overproduction of misfolded proteins). But these aspects need to be further explored in experimental studies, in order to draw more consistent conclusions.

Brain/Hypothalamic Immune Receptors and Metabolic Syndrome

The mechanisms that have been described above do not require activation of specific receptors to be triggered. But, together with them, some immune receptor-mediated pathways can also be activated in hypothalamic inflammatory cascades contributing to MetS in overnutrition-induced dysregulations. In this context, toll-like receptors' (TLRs) activation has captured researchers' attention, in recent years.

TLRs are a class of membrane-bound proteins that play an important role in the innate immune defense, recognizing structurally conserved molecular patterns derived from "nonself" molecules. They are mainly expressed in sentinel cells, like macrophages and dendritic cells, and also hypothalamic neurons and glia cells have these receptors at the surface, meaning that they can locally mediate innate immune response to stimuli coming from the periphery or being produced at the site [31]. Overnutrition can be an environmental stimulus leading to the activation of some isoforms of TLRs. In fact, TLR1, 2, 4, and 6 are responsive to extracellular lipids, as demonstrated in studies using adipocytes, macrophages, and myocytes [32]. Specifically at the hypothalamic level, TLR4 has been shown to be activated in response to lipid excess [33], and, after its inhibition, it was possible to demonstrate, in mice, a significant prevention of some overnutrition-induced metabolic problems, such as leptin and insulin resistance and weight gain. The inhibition of TLR4 signaling specifically in mice brain was able to reproduce the protective effects of a systemic TLR4 deficiency [34].

In addition to TLRs, also cytokine receptors may be implicated in the pathogenesis of central dysfunctions in MetS. Actually, the presence of cytokines in several peripheral tissues and also in circulation is a prominent feature of metabolic diseases. The hypothalamus has a permissive blood-brain barrier around the mediobasal region and is particularly sensitive to circulating cytokines, which may easily activate local receptors and potentiate on-site production of the same kind of substances, sustaining and enhancing inflammation [35]. Tumor necrosis factor alpha (TNF-α) is one of the cytokines with more studies supporting its role in the development of MetS components. Central administration of low doses of this pro-inflammatory molecule replicates metabolic inflammation and, thus, enhances eating and decreases energy consumption, leading to obesity and arterial hypertension [36]. Studies with transgenic animals point in the same direction: genetically deficient mice (either to TNF-α or its receptor) are protected from the development of insulin resistance and obesity under overnutrition conditions [37]. On the other hand, interleukin-6 (IL-6) and IL-10 that share anti-inflammatory properties were found to be linked to the benefits of physical exercise by reducing hypothalamic inflammation [38].

Taken together, these data support the role that the immune system may have (at least through TLRs and cytokine receptors) in the development of central metabolic dysfunctions leading to MetS and related disorders. But, naturally, further studies are needed to better characterize the dialogue between immune cells and molecules and the brain, in the context of overnutrition.

IKKβ/NF-κB Signaling in Overnutrition-Induced Inflammation

IκB kinase β (IKKβ) and nuclear factor-κB (NF-κB) make part of a relevant pro-inflammatory pathway in mammalian cells, exerting a key role in innate immune responses. In a resting state, NF-κB is located in the cytoplasm assuming an inactive form, which results from the masking provided by a complex group of little molecules. After contact with immune stimuli, IKKβ is activated via a receptor-mediated pathway and phosphorylates the blocker, resulting on its ubiquitination and subsequent degradation. NF-κB is released, enters the nucleus, and starts to induce the transcription of several genes that are responsible for a large number of cellular processes: inflammation, immunity, proliferation, apoptosis, and senescence [39].

Research in the last 10 years has linked IKKβ/NF-κB pathway activation to several metabolic disorders related to overnutrition, and one of the most prominent features of the activation of this pathway is that it contributes to a low-grade and chronic inflammation, impairing normal intracellular signaling and metabolic physiology. CNS neurons (and particularly those contained in the hypothalamus) are very sensitive to this metabolic inflammation, but the trigger leading to hypothalamic NF-κB activation is not entirely clear, so far. Nevertheless, intracellular oxidative stress and mitochondrial dysfunction seem to be key elements in the activation of this pro-inflammatory pathway under overnutrition and without any specific receptor activation [9]. ROS may induce phosphorylation of NF-κB masking system (mainly – but not exclusively – via IκBα), removing its physiological inhibition [40], and, alternatively, they can also inactivate (by oxidation) other proteins involved in controlling several steps of this pathway, such as IKK phosphatases and PTEN (phosphatase and tensin homologue, an Akt phosphatase) [41]. In peripheral tissues, the role of NF-κB activation by oxidative stress has been linked to some MetS-related diseases, such as diabetes, stroke, myocardial infarction, and atherosclerosis [42]. However, in the CNS, the potential link between NF-κB activation and oxidative stress in mediating central metabolic dysregulations in MetS is not so clear, deserving naturally further research. Still, there are some data coming from different studies that may support this hypothesis: (1) as it was previously said, overnutrition is an environmental stimulus capable of inducing oxidative stress in different types of tissues and the CNS is not an exception [12–15]; (2) NF-κB activation has been shown to be produced by oxidative stress in neurons or glial cells [43, 44]; (3) central glucose or lipid excess has been demonstrated to activate hypothalamic NF-κB [20, 34]; and (4) inhibition of ROS production and suppression of NF-κB activation by sirtuin 1, a histone deacetylase, has been shown to protect against aging and atherosclerosis, a condition frequently associated with MetS [45]. All these data support the notion that the relationship between oxidative stress and NF-κB is more or less like a vicious cycle: ROS may contribute to NF-κB pathway activation, which, in turn, induces ROS-producing enzymes, enhancing refractoriness that is often associated with overnutrition-induced metabolic dysfunction.

Endoplasmic reticulum stress has also been investigated in this context. Several evidences are coming from different groups favoring its role on the activation of the NF-κB inflammatory pathway and this has been well addressed in the CNS. Recent studies demonstrated that a high-fat diet induces endoplasmic reticulum stress and IKKβ/NF-κB activation in mice hypothalamus and also that, while feeding mice with a normal chow diet, the same pro-inflammatory pathway is activated if the animals are injected concomitantly with an endoplasmic reticulum stress inducer [20]. In the same line of evidence, the infusion of an endoplasmic reticulum stress inhibitor directly to the third ventricle suppresses the activation of hypothalamic NF-κB by a high-fat diet [20]. But, as was the case of oxidative stress, also the development of endoplasmic reticulum stress appears to be dependent, to some extent, on IKKβ/NF-κB pathway activity, because it was shown that no hypothalamic endoplasmic reticulum stress is produced (using high-fat diet feeding and chemical stress inducers as stimuli) if a previous central IKKβ/NF-κB inhibition is performed [20, 46]. Finally, it is worth to notice that endoplasmic reticulum stress can also promote inflammation via induction of oxidative stress, and, given this, it is not difficult to imagine a model where factors contributing to the final result reciprocally enhance and promote each other, making that result (in this case, central metabolic dysregulations) more expressive and clear.

An additional element playing a role in developing metabolic dysfunction in overnutrition-induced conditions is, as previously stated, autophagy defect. A connection between this defect and NF-κB activation in CNS was very recently proved. Mice with knockdown of Atg7 (autophagy-related protein 7) were demonstrated to have a hypothalamic autophagy defect and a concomitant activation of IKKβ/NF-κB pathway, exacerbating the development of obesity (under high-fat diet feeding) and metabolic comorbidities [30]. The relationship that directly links hypothalamic autophagy defect and NF-κB-induced inflammation was stressed by the observation that, suppressing IKKβ in hypothalamic cells, it was possible to halt the effects of autophagy defect on central metabolic control [30].

The close link between IKKβ/NF-κB signaling, TLRs, and cytokine receptor pathways deserves also to be highlighted. In experimental studies, it was shown that overnutrition activates TLR4 signaling, which played a crucial role in activating IKKβ/NF-κB pathway, leading to leptin resistance, glucose intolerance, and weight gain [33, 34]. That activation is, at least in an early phase, dependent on the myeloid differentiation factor 88 (MyD88), because the brain-specific deletion of this factor has a negative impact on the activation of the IKKβ/NF-κB pathway via TLR4 [34]. In addition to its role on the activation of pro-inflammatory kinase pathways, TLR4 has also been shown to potentiate intracellular endoplasmic reticulum stress, which contributes to prove that it also plays a strategic role in overnutrition-induced inflammation [18].

In the same line of thought, cytokine receptor signaling is also associated with NF-κB activation, but the biologic effect resulting of this activation seems to be cell type dependent: in hypothalamic AgRP neurons cytokines primarily lead to energy imbalance and obesity, while in POMC neurons they are mainly associated with the development of glucose intolerance and hypertension [7, 46]. Central administration of IL-4 leads to microglial activation and, thus, promotes hypothalamic inflammation resulting in weight gain, this net result being abolished by administering an IKKβ inhibitor [47]. This implies that glial cells may also be involved in causing central dysregulation of metabolism in MetS, possibly via cytokine production that exert their effect by a paracrine mechanism. However, this interaction between neurons and glia, in the context of MetS-related disorders, needs further research to become clear. All the knowledge currently available related to inflammatory activity mediated by NF-κB in CNS, in MetS patients, is probably a drop in the ocean of the

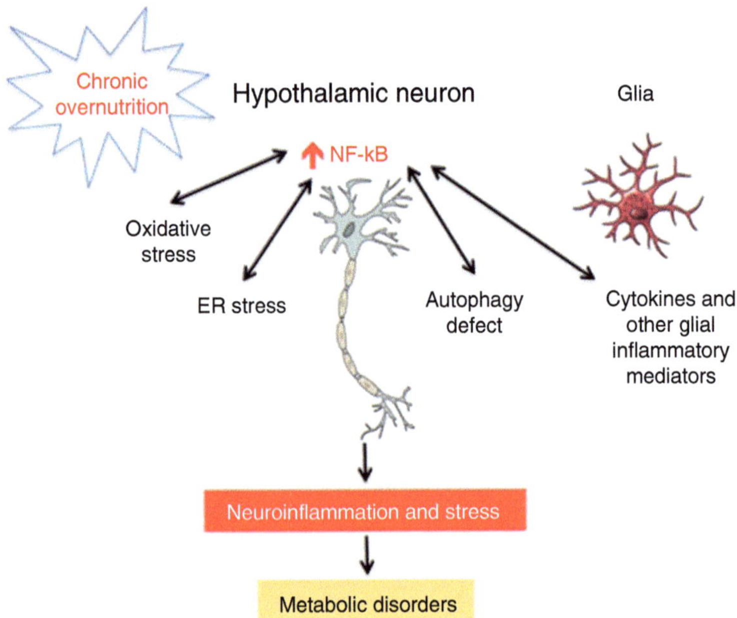

Fig. 7.1 Role of hypothalamic neuroinflammation in metabolic disorders. In the context of chronic overnutrition, there is an activation of the IKKβ/NF-κB pro-inflammatory pathway, mainly produced by an oxidative stress, by an endoplasmic reticulum (ER) stress, and by a defective autophagy machinery. Glia-neuron inflammatory cross talk is also relevant, and these abnormalities, collectively, lead to hypothalamic neuronal dysfunction and to the development of a spectrum of metabolic disorders

pathophysiological mechanisms related to disease, yet. In recent years this knowledge has expanded very significantly, but the margin for improvement is still enormous [48]. Figure 7.1 summarizes some of the concepts presented.

Neurodegeneration and Neurogenesis in Metabolic Syndrome

The relevance of the hypothalamus in the development of MetS, for all that has been said, is unquestionable. Indeed, classical studies showed that the ablation of some ventral nuclei causes overeating and obesity in animals, while lesions produced at a more lateral level lead to anorexia and weight loss. Although scientifically relevant, these data do not explain the pathophysiology and the mechanisms implicated in clinical outcomes. However, recent studies have been showing a connection between neurodegeneration and the development of metabolic disturbances, such as T2D and obesity [49]: in the first place, using adult mice fed with a high-fat diet, it was possible to show a reduction in the number of hypothalamic POMC neurons [49]; and second, chronic overnutrition was shown to be responsible for increasing apoptosis of mature and newborn neurons and neural stem cells in the hypothalamus, this situation being to some extent reversed by caloric restriction [49, 50]. This is especially interesting, taking into account that studies on postnatal hypothalamic development have been able to show that neurons in the ARC undergo postnatal turnover, even in adulthood [50]. Real clinical implications of such an observation are still insufficiently studied, but these data are important to counteract the old dogma which looks at the CNS as a static system in which neuronal damage is absolutely irreversible and irreparable.

Inflammation seems to be the leading cause of hypothalamic neurodegeneration in MetS-related disorders, such as obesity and T2D, and this is a common background shared with typical neurodegenerative diseases. As it was previously discussed, IKKβ/NF-κB pathway is critically involved in the development of hypothalamic damage in metabolic dysfunctions and in neurodegeneration itself, but there are several unanswered questions in this area that make it very attractive to future research. Indeed, the role of inflammation in promoting neurogenesis and repair in metabolic disturbances is not yet fully understood.

It is well established that adult mammalian brains contain multipotent neural stem cells that have the intrinsic ability to generate and to differentiate into several cell types in the CNS, from neurons to oligodendrocytes [51]. These adult stem cells might be able to be involved in adult neurogenesis and in maintaining brain plasticity in response to intrinsic and extrinsic stress. They are predominantly localized in the subventricular zone of the forebrain lateral ventricle and in the subgranular zone of the hippocampal dentate gyrus [52]. The research made in the last decade has proved that the hypothalamus of adult mice has neurogenic activity in basal conditions [53] and after stimulation [54]. More recently, it has been shown that, using a mouse model with genetically induced degeneration of neurons expressing AgRP, de novo hypothalamic neurogenesis exists, leading to the development of new leptin-responsive AgRP neurons [55]. In addition, neurons contained in the ARC of adult mice were demonstrated to have intrinsic physiological turnover activity [50], but it was also discovered that IKKβ/NF-κB pathway activation stimulates an apoptotic program impairing the survival of hypothalamic neural stem cells and that turnover capacity [49]. Thus, it is critical to note that IKKβ/NF-κB-mediated inflammation not only affects neurohormonal pathways and signaling axis in hypothalamic neurons, which are relevant for regulating metabolic physiology, but also hampers neurogenesis and repair mechanisms, leading to the development of metabolic diseases. All this knowledge has been raising a huge scientific interest in hypothalamic repair properties and mechanisms and, logically, in their role for the development of systemic metabolic disorders [56]. Consolidation of this knowledge may have a huge impact on future design of pharmacological and cellular therapies for MetS.

Therapeutic Applications

The concept of brain stress in MetS is a relatively recent establishment and, therefore, the amount of mechanistic studies conducted specifically for developing new potential therapeutic agents is still scarce. However, the recognition of the deleterious role of IKKβ/NF-κB pro-inflammatory pathway activation in hypothalamic cells has contributed to the design of some experiments showing that its inhibition effectively protects against metabolic disorders. Several strategies were used in animal models: (1) pharmacologic inhibition of hypothalamic IKKβ [57]; (2) brain-specific deletion of the same enzyme [20], of one of the signaling effectors of the IKKβ/NF-κB pathway, the SOCS3 protein (suppressor of cytokine signaling-3) [58], or of TLR4 signaling adaptor MyD88 [34]; and (3) whole-body genetic deficiency of TLR4 [33] or NF-κB subunit p50 [59]. Data coming from studies in humans are much more scarce, but there are some reports in the literature that it is worth to consider here. In a retrospective case-control study, acetylsalicylic acid used as an anti-inflammatory drug was shown to promote weight loss in T2D patients [60]. Also, rimonabant (a drug specifically developed for weight loss but already withdrawn from the market) was responsible for a systemic decrease of inflammatory response [61].

Improving endoplasmic reticulum stress can also constitute itself as a therapeutic target in MetS and that was achieved in obese mice by inducing genetic expression of some UPR components and chaperone proteins or administering a pharmacologic endoplasmic reticulum stress inhibitor, such as tauroursodeoxycholic acid (TUDCA) [62]. In fact, this organelle-specific therapy demonstrated to have some measurable biologic effects in humans. TUDCA was able to improve liver and muscle insulin sensitivity in obese subjects [63], and stavudine, a drug with antioxidant properties, was demonstrated to increase muscle insulin sensitivity in humans [64].

Finally, considering MetS-associated CVD, many clinical and epidemiological studies have been done to demonstrate the therapeutic potential of anti-cellular stress drugs. Vitamin E (which has a well-known antioxidant activity), coenzyme Q10, α-lipoic acid, and α-L-carnitine are some examples of substances acting as protectors of myocardial dysfunction, as oxidation-resistant low-density lipoprotein production enhancers and as systolic blood pressure improvers in patients with coronary heart disease [65]. It is known that overnutrition-related metabolic inflammation in the hypothalamus (particularly in POMC neurons) may contribute to the development of arterial hypertension, at least in obese mice [66]. However, this knowledge is so recent that it is still premature to speculate about any therapy which may have an antihypertensive activity and that potentially may have its mechanism of action contained in this pathway.

Indeed, despite the exciting discoveries that have been made over the past years, connecting metabolic inflammation with the brain (particularly with the hypothalamus) and with MetS-related conditions is still a great challenge and many important questions still remain to be answered and to find some support coming from experimental environments. Current understandings of the central inflammatory mechanisms that mediate MetS and its related disorders are still in a very early stage. And this is even more striking considering the possibility of therapeutic intervention on these dysfunctional mechanisms. However, this is a field of great clinical significance, and major research campaigns are being implemented to effectively translate this scientific knowledge into novel and effective treatments against MetS.

Systemic Metabolic Dysfunction in Neurodegenerative Disorders

Alzheimer's Disease

Alzheimer's disease (AD) is the most common cause of dementia. This neurodegenerative disorder has a characteristic neuropathology, which consists of senile plaques (aggregates of amyloid β [Aβ] protein surrounded by damaged neuronal processes and reactive glia) and neurofibrillary tangles (intraneuronal aggregates of hyperphosphorylated tau protein) leading to loss of synapses and neuronal death.

The neuroinflammatory processes underlying AD pathology have been the subject of research for the last years, with important advances in the understanding of the intricate interaction between CNS resident cells and the systemic immune response. Microglia has arisen as the main character involved in communication between local and systemic inflammation. The major regulator of this microglial priming is the composition of the CNS microenvironment. Local neuronal damage and accumulation of misfolded proteins (such as seen in AD) can reduce inhibition or directly activate microglia, which produce a maladaptive response and perpetuate neuronal death. Aging, the major risk factor for developing AD, is characterized by a chronic low-grade systemic inflammation appearing as a result of the decline in the function of the adaptive immune system and persistence of an intact innate immune system (upregulation of Th1 pro-inflammatory response and relative decline in Th2 anti-inflammatory response). With increasing age, microglia also adopts an activated phenotype.

ApoE4, the best established genetic risk factor for developing sporadic late-onset AD [67, 68], besides its important role in lipid transport [68], has also been associated with the degree of microglial activation in response to Aβ depositions. In AD, the blood-brain barrier (BBB) becomes leaky because of Aβ accumulation along the brain blood vessels (cerebral amyloid angiopathy), causing associated vascular inflammation and impaired clearance of Aβ across the BBB [69]. Acute (e.g., infection) and chronic systemic inflammation (e.g., atherosclerosis, obesity, and diabetes) have been held responsible for the microglial priming and polarization to a sustained neurodegenerative phenotype as well [70].

We will now refer to the systemic inflammatory and metabolic dysfunction that could perpetuate this neurodegenerative process within the CNS and briefly comment on novel therapies with an emphasis on modifiable lifestyle changes that could prevent cognitive impairment or improve cognitive performance.

A number of pro- and anti-inflammatory cytokines have been associated with AD and risk of overall dementia, including TNF-α, IL-1, IL-6, IL-7, IL-10, IL-15, and IL-18, although their relationship with plausible biological explanations are still matter of research. Acute inflammatory states (e.g., infection) have demonstrated the connection between circulating pro-inflammatory cytokines and the development of behavioral and psychological symptoms ("sickness illness") among patients with AD, demonstrating that raised TNF-α and IL-6, but not C-reactive protein (CRP), were associated with an approximately twofold increased frequency of neuropsychiatric sickness behavior in AD patients, independent of the development of delirium [71]. On the other hand, one of the most studied chronic inflammatory states that have been associated with the risk of AD and other dementias is the MetS. Association between MetS and cognitive performance is dependent of age. In younger adults, MetS increases the risk of dementia, but in older adults over the age of 75, MetS is associated with better cognitive performance and reduced risk of dementia [72, 73].

When lipid consumption exceeds the metabolic capacity of macrophages, lipotoxicity and accumulation of metabolites within adipose and non-adipose tissue compartments such as oxidized LDL, free fatty acids (FFA), cholesterol, and ceramide, among others, induce chronic inflammation by promoting macrophage infiltration and activation [74, 75]. Activated macrophages produce excessive secretion of pro-inflammatory cytokines (e.g., TNF-α, IL-1β, monocyte chemoattractant protein-1 [MCP1], CRP), inducing insulin resistance by interfering with insulin/insulin-like growth factor 1 (IGF-1) signaling, causing increased circulating FFA and reduced glucose uptake. Insulin is one of the most consistent components of the MetS that could predict cognitive performance. In healthy controls, higher insulin levels predicted more rapid decline in attention and verbal memory over 2 years, in opposition to early AD patients in whom higher insulin levels predicted better cognitive performance [76]. Insulin affects neuronal performance and cognition by regulating ion channels, neurotransmitter receptors, and synaptic transmission in the AD-diseased brain [77]. It provides direct negative feedback to hypothalamic nuclei that control whole-body energy and glucose homeostasis, and dietary fat is able to induce hypothalamic inflammation resulting in insulin/leptin resistance [78]. Insulin dysregulation has also been associated to reduce brain glucose utilization, neurofibrillary tangle formation, and Aβ aggregation by insulin-degrading enzyme inhibition in AD patients [77]. Therefore, systemic inflammation and insulin resistance may represent convergent mechanisms through which comorbid metabolic disorders promote the development of AD [78].

There has been special interest in the role of obesity and adipokines and the risk of dementia. Obesity is also characterized by a chronic low-inflammatory state mediated by the production of IL-1 and IL-6. The hippocampus has been shown to be especially vulnerable to IL-6, affecting brain functions such as synaptic plasticity and neurogenesis, disrupting learning and memory processes. Higher levels of plasma IL-6 are also correlated with lower hippocampal gray matter volume. Adipokines or adipocytokines are signaling molecules secreted by peripheral white adipose tissue, and they have been associated with dysregulation of nutrient utilization, inflammation, endothelial dysfunction, hypertension, and atherogenesis and have also been held responsible for the link between obesity and dementia. For example, leptin has been shown to affect hypothalamic function, learning, and memory processes controlled by the hippocampus and to regulate energy expenditure and food intake [79], and adiponectin is involved in the modulation of inflammatory responses, decreasing the expression of inflammatory cytokines (TNF-α), increasing the expression of anti-inflammatory molecules (IL-10, IL-1 receptor antagonist), and decreasing activation of the pro-inflammatory NF-κB signal pathway. Adiponectin also modulates energy expenditure in the CNS (modifying sensitivity to insulin in the brain) and at the periphery, and it regulates food intake and several other metabolic processes. It modulates memory and cognitive impairment and contributes to the dysregulated glucose metabolism and mitochondrial dysfunction observed in AD [77].

Plasma cholesterol could also be a factor involved in the production of Aβ and in the development of neuropsychiatric symptoms in AD. Triglyceride levels have been correlated with depression [80], and it has been described a "longevity phenotype" characterized by large LDL and HDL serum levels, associated with homozygosity for a genetic variant of cholesterol ester transfer protein (CETP) and preservation of cognitive function [81]. Some authors have also correlated neuropsychiatric symptoms with biomarkers of cardiovascular risk (total cholesterol being the strongest marker in males) and with biomarkers of systemic inflammation (IL-15 being the strongest marker in women) [80].

All the aforementioned risk factors are common between AD and vascular dementia, and some data from large cardiovascular cohorts have shed some light on the impact of biomarkers of systemic inflammation in the development of AD and cognitive impairment. In the Rotterdam study, elderly subjects with higher levels of α1-antichymotrypsin and IL-6 had an increased risk of incident dementia and AD [82]. In the Framingham study, subjects with the highest production of IL-1β and TNF-α had an increased risk of developing incident AD [83]. Finally, in a population-based study, higher levels of baseline TNF-α and intermittent increases triggered by acute factors (like infection) were associated with a more rapid progression of cognitive decline [84].

Although there is a better understanding of the mechanisms underlying the association between systemic inflammation and neurodegeneration in AD, many therapeutic approaches have failed to demonstrate real benefits in preventing or slowing the progression of the disease. Long-term nonsteroidal anti-inflammatory drugs (NSAIDs) could have a protective effect against the development of AD, probably due to the regulation of cyclooxygenase-1 (COX-1) and cyclooxygenase-2 (COX-2) activity [85] or regulating microglial reactivity [86], although prospective clinical trials have failed to demonstrate therapeutic benefit with the use of naproxen, celecoxib, or rofecoxib [87].

In a recent meta-analysis exploring the benefit of statins in dementia, Wong et al. found that statin use could have a beneficial role in AD patients (RR: 0.70, 95 % CI [0.60, 0.83]) [88]. Some of this protective role could be in part secondary to lower levels of cholesterol, although their anti-inflammatory effect (activation of heme-oxygenase/biliverdin reductase system and inhibition of isoprenylation of small GTP-binding proteins) and other pleiotropic properties may also be involved [89].

Pilot trials with intranasal insulin administration suggested promising cognitive improvement and modulation of Aβ deposition in patients with mild cognitive impairment (MCI) and AD [90, 91]. Antioxidant therapy (e.g., coenzyme Q, vitamin E, vitamin C, and α-lipoid acid) has demonstrated significant decrease in cerebrospinal fluid F2 isoprostane (biomarker of oxidative damage) with no long-term clinical benefits. More recently, immunotherapy and inhibition of TNF-α is being investigated as a potential candidate for AD treatment. Some studies suggest that TNF-α haplotype could be a disease-modifier gene in patients genetically predisposed to AD, and there have been some reports of anti-TNF agents (e.g., infliximab, etanercept, pentoxifylline) that have shown some improvement in the cognitive performance of AD patients, although definitive clinical trials are still lacking [92].

Finally, diet and exercise are among the lifestyle changes associated with reducing biomarkers of systemic inflammation and showing promising results on neurodegeneration. High-calorie Western diet, rich in saturated fatty acids and cholesterol, is associated with the development of AD-like cognitive impairment [93]. Animal models suggest that such diets could cause increased amyloidosis and altered synaptic plasticity and behavior, and high-fat diet and excessive sucrose intake have also been shown to enhance tau pathology in mice [70]. On the contrary, many studies suggest that adherence to a Mediterranean diet may be associated with a reduced risk of developing AD. Some authors have found a correlation between diet and levels of blood inflammatory biomarkers, but others have failed to determine whether this protective factor is involved with inflammatory or metabolic pathways, probably due to different experimental and statistical approaches [94]. Exercise promotes better sleep and cardiorespiratory fitness, reduces obesity, and modulates cortisol levels. Aerobic exercise training has shown several benefits, such as the following: (1) to improve resting cerebrovascular reactivity to hypercapnia; (2) to reduce arterial pressure; (3) to decrease total cholesterol and triglycerides blood levels; (4) to lower body mass index (BMI); (5) to promote a better glycemic control; (6) to increase IGF-1 levels and regional brain volume in older adults, specifically at the hippocampus level; and (7) to promote brain neurogenesis and to reduce chronic low-grade inflammation (decreasing TNF-α and IL-6), and this could be a link between exercise and prevention of AD and overall dementia [95, 96].

In summary, although aging and apoE4 status appears to be the greatest and most studied and validated non-modifiable risk factors for developing sporadic AD, systemic inflammation and cardiometabolic risk factors are probably the link between AD and vascular dementia and could be a promising therapeutic target for novel treatment approaches and for early prevention strategies, including exercise and healthy lifestyle changes.

Multiple Sclerosis

Multiple sclerosis (MS) is a chronic immune-mediated disease characterized by acute and chronic inflammation within the CNS, associated to focal demyelination (MS plaques) and progressive neuroaxonal degeneration. It is the leading cause of nontraumatic neurological disability among young adults, and although the precise etiology is still unknown, genetic predisposition associated to environmental factors (low levels of vitamin D, smoking, infections) has been proposed to be the trigger of a pathogenic immune response against CNS antigens, developing and perpetuating MS distinct inflammatory processes [97, 98].

The complete understanding of the immunopathogenesis of the disease is out of the scope of this chapter, but, briefly, cellular and humoral components of the immune system are compromised in MS pathology: the innate immune system is involved in several steps, including the activation of myelin-reactive T lymphocytes by antigen-presenting cells (including B lymphocytes) at the periphery and the development of membrane attack complexes within the CNS; the adaptive immune system is also affected, where T cells that specifically recognize myelin fragments induce tissue damage and contribute to lesion formation. Active MS plaques are characterized by T cell, macrophage and activated microglial infiltration, and the presence of immune mediators, including adhesion molecules, chemokines, and cytokines [99], which are responsible for generating BBB leakage, destruction of myelin sheaths, oligodendrocyte damage and cell death, glial scar formation, inflammatory infiltrates and axonal damage, and, at the end, neuronal loss [100]. Neuronal and axonal degeneration in MS is a slow process that is probably initiated by acute lymphocytic infiltration and subsequently driven by chronically smoldering and diffuse parenchymal myeloid and meningeal lymphocytic inflammation [97]. As in AD, the microglia also plays a key role in the inflammation-induced neurodegeneration occurring during both acute and chronic stages of MS. These cells have been associated to the formation of cortical lesions in MS, and they also play an important role in the promotion of neuroprotection, downregulation of inflammation, and stimulation of tissue repair. As explained above, the microglia undergoes changes in morphology and function with normal aging, resulting in a decline of its ability to repair CNS damage, making axons and neurons more vulnerable as people grow older [101]. The microglia is also known to be affected by acute and chronic systemic inflammation, responding to circulating cytokines and producing immune mediators that lead to tissue damage, which prolongs the neurodegenerative-perpetuating phenotype of these cells [102].

Although local persistent inflammation within the CNS (e.g., lymphoid leptomeningeal follicles) is probably associated with sustained disability, systemic chronic inflammation has also been held responsible for the progression of neurodegenerative processes among these patients, with a new target for novel therapeutic interventions waiting to be confirmed. Furthermore, the presence of systemic inflammation and increased cardiometabolic risk among MS patients has also been a motive of research. We will now refer to the biomarkers of cardiometabolic risk and inflammation that have been associated with this disease.

In a study of 833 clinically stable patients, Martins et al. found differences in serum Th1 cytokine concentrations (increased IFN-γ and IL-2) and monokines (an increase in TNF-α and IL-1β and a decrease in IL-8, a neutrophil attractant) and no differences in IL-6 levels between MS patients and healthy controls. Anti-inflammatory Th2 cytokine levels were also found to be different (higher levels of IL-4 and IL-13 in MS patients, with no differences in IL-5 concentrations) and these changes were not related to the MS clinical phenotype. The increase of both pro- and anti-inflammatory cytokines in patients with MS seems to be consistent with the simultaneous inflammatory and restorative processes underlying the disease [99].

Chronic inflammation is a relevant factor for the development of atherosclerosis, contributing to the increased risk of overall vascular risk and added disability among patients with MS. There have been contradictory findings when evaluating vascular risk in patients with MS, although it seems that these patients are in higher risk of developing vascular disease than the general population [103]. In a cohort of male veterans with MS, the subset of people aged 50 years or older was found to be at higher risk of developing T2D, hypertension, hypercholesterolemia, coronary heart disease, and stroke than general population [104]. Other studies report higher risks of stroke and cerebrovascular disease, especially during the first years after MS diagnosis and among young and middle-aged patients and increased risk of venous thromboembolism, including deep vein thrombosis and pulmonary embolism, but lower prevalence of coronary artery disease including myocardial infarction [105], with special attention in women [106]. In 2010, Marrie et al. showed that vascular comorbidities were present in more than 50 % of patients (37 % had hypercholesterolemia, 30 % arterial hypertension, 7 % heart disease, 6 % T2D, and 2 % peripheral vascular disease). Vascular comorbidities at any time during the disease course were associated with a 1.5-fold increase of the risk of ambulatory disability [107].

Serum lipid levels' dysregulation has been described to be present among MS patients, who frequently show increased levels of triglycerides and oxidized LDL and reduced concentrations of HDL, with an interesting correlation between oxidized-LDL levels and the expanded disability status scale (EDSS) score, as reported by Palavra et al. [108]. The North American Research Committee on Multiple Sclerosis (NARCOMS) registry study reported that 37 % of patients with MS suffered from hypercholesterolemia, which was a higher value than that coming from the general population [103], although some studies reported figures with a much lower prevalence. The brain is believed to be particularly susceptible to lipid dysregulation and oxidative damage, due to its composition with high content of lipids and high oxygen consumption [109]. Associations between HDL or triglyceride levels and brain contrast-enhancing lesions in clinically isolated syndrome (CIS) or early MS patients have also been found [110], but further research is needed to confirm these data.

In this matter, statins have emerged in the MS field, calling attention to their pleiotropic immunomodulatory and anti-inflammatory effects, independent of their effect on lipid profile. Although several clinical trials have taken place testing the role of statins as monotherapy or in combination with disease-modifying therapies, there have been some conflicting results (summarized in a recent meta-analysis by Ciurleo et al.) [111]. This is probably in part because of diverse drug regimens and different methodological and statistical models used, including results with favorable outcomes (such as reduction of gadolinium-enhancing lesions, reduction of relapse rate, reduction of brain atrophy and disability progression, as it was recently shown in a study involving secondary progressive MS patients [112]), as opposed to no significant reduction in relapse rate or disease progression or even increased magnetic resonance imaging (MRI) and clinical disease activity and antagonism of interferon-beta function in some cohorts [111, 113]. Further investigation and reproducible results should be awaited before the regular use of statins in MS patients in daily clinical practice, as highlighted by Sena et al. [114–116]. Although there are well-known adverse effects associated to the use of this family of drugs, it appears that they will achieve an acceptable safety and tolerability profile [111].

As in AD, obesity and adipocytokines have also been related to MS. In the best-known animal model of the disease (experimental autoimmune encephalitis [EAE]), caloric restriction was associated to higher levels of serum adiponectin (anti-inflammatory adipokine) and reduced susceptibility and severity of EAE. In addition, leptin, a pro-inflammatory adipokine, appears to be a requisite for EAE induction [117]. Accordingly, leptin-deficient mice have been shown to present myelin with an abnormal biochemical composition and also a decrease in CNS myelination, thus contributing to make these animals resistant to the disease [6, 117].

In recent studies, women with MS have been shown to have higher BMI than recommended by the World Health Organization (50 % being overweighed, of which 50 % were obese), but this is not different from higher BMI seen in normal controls [103]. Furthermore, an interesting association between obesity (especially in childhood and adolescence) and an increased risk for developing MS has been observed, although this association was only significant for females, showing a dose-dependent relationship [118]. Other theories associating obesity and MS include the relationship between the coexistence of HLA-DRB1*15 and obesity (increased risk for developing MS, OR=3) or the absence of HLA-A*02 and presence of obesity (increased risk for developing MS, OR=15) [119]. The association between obesity, lipid profile, and levels of serum vitamin D has also been reported, stressing that higher levels of vitamin D are associated with a reduced risk of MS in early adulthood and that total body fat is inversely related to the levels of circulating 15-hidroxy-vitamin D [120]. This vitamin is known to produce immunomodulatory and antioxidant effects, regulates the expression of cyclooxygenases, interferes with transcription factors such as NF-κB, regulates activation of signaling cascades (such as MAP kinases, among others), and targets a myriad of cell types such as monocytes/macrophages, dendritic cells, and B and T lymphocytes. All of the above have given rise to a large amount of studies evaluating the effect of vitamin D supplementation in MS patients with promising results [120].

Glucose metabolism could also be impaired in patients with MS and higher risks of T2D are reported in literature [103]. The association between T2D and higher disability has also been shown in the NARCOMS cohort [107]. In a recent study of

110 patients with MS and 175 healthy controls, a higher proportion of insulin resistance among MS patients (40 % vs. 21 %, OR = 2.48) was found, and those patients with insulin resistance showed higher EDSS scores, IL-6 and IL-17 levels, as well as markers of oxidative stress than MS patients with normal glucose metabolism. In a multivariate analysis, EDSS score was also associated with central adiposity and BMI, and hyperinsulinemia was related with cognitive impairment in MS [121].

More recently, in laboratorial studies, it has been shown that salt modulates the differentiation of human and mouse Th17 cells. Also, mice fed with a high-sodium diet were reported to develop a more aggressive form of EAE, calling attention to the deleterious role that excessive salt consumption can have on disease development. In a study recently published by Farez et al., the authors were able to demonstrate that high-sodium intake in patients diagnosed with MS is associated with an increase in relapse rate and in the chance of developing new T2 lesions on the MRI [122].

In summary, although local inflammatory processes within the CNS have been the main research target for the last years in patients with MS (leading to the development of more than ten different disease-modifying drugs approved for the relapsing-remitting form of the disease by the date of this review), progressive MS and the underlying neurodegenerative processes of the disease are still a dry field for pharmacotherapeutics. Controlling systemic inflammation and cardiometabolic risk

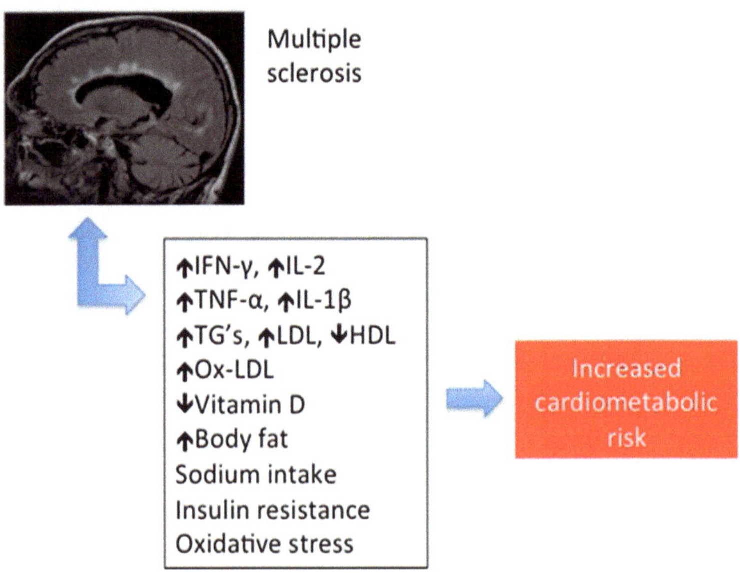

Fig. 7.2 Main aspects that contribute to an increased cardiometabolic risk in patients with multiple sclerosis. *IFN-γ* interferon gamma, *IL* interleukin, *TNF-α* tumor necrosis factor alpha, *TGs* triglycerides, *LDL* low-density lipoprotein, *HDL* high-density lipoprotein, *Ox-LDL* oxidized-low-density lipoprotein. Arrows pointing up represent an increase and arrows pointing down represent a decrease

factors (the most relevant players are summarized in Fig. 7.2) could be a useful and cost-effective therapeutic strategy and a novel approach to prevent further disability accumulation among MS patients, with indisputable benefits in the general well-being.

Other Neurodegenerative Disorders

Parkinson's disease (PD) has also been a subject of research, considering possible associations between a genetic predisposition and exposure to environmental, toxic, or cardiometabolic inflammation triggers. Probably, the activation of microglial cells within the CNS, induced by systemic low-grade inflammation such as seen in AD, also plays a key role in progressive and irreversible neurodegenerative processes underlying PD. Increased levels of pro-inflammatory mediators such as TNF-α, IL-1β, IL-6, ROS, and eicosanoids have been found in postmortem analysis of the substantia nigra of PD patients and in animal models of the disease [123]. Similar findings have been described in depression, chronic fatigue syndrome, schizophrenia, and Huntington's and prion diseases [70, 124, 125].

In conclusion, the association between systemic inflammation and neurodegeneration is probably some sort of a common ground among many disorders, more than a disease-specific process of each particular illness. Possibly, finding the distinctive trigger or an individual inflammatory biomarker characteristic for each disease would generate an effective therapeutic approach to stop the development of neuroaxonal loss and disability accumulation. Or, perhaps, fighting against common systemic inflammatory processes, such as MetS, obesity, or low blood levels of vitamin D, will change, in the near future, the way we look at these high-burden conditions.

References

1. Nguyen DM, El-Serag HB. The epidemiology of obesity. Gastroenterol Clin North Am. 2010;39(1):1–7.
2. Yoon KH, Lee JU, Kim JW, et al. Epidemic obesity and type 2 diabetes in Asia. Lancet. 2006;368(9548):1681–8.
3. Abelson P, Kennedy D. The obesity epidemic. Science. 2004;304(5676):1413.
4. Kaur J. A comprehensive review on metabolic syndrome. Cardiol Res Pract. 2014;2014:943162.
5. Lumeng CN, Saltiel AR. Inflammatory links between obesity and metabolic disease. J Clin Invest. 2011;121(6):2111–7.
6. Sena A, Sarliève LL, Rebel G. Brain myelin of genetically obese mice. J Neurol Sci. 1985;68:233–44.
7. Purkayastha S, Cai D. Neuroinflammatory basis of metabolic syndrome. Mol Metab. 2013;2(4):356–63.
8. López M, Tovar S, Vázquez MJ, Williams LM, Diéguez C. Peripheral tissue-brain interactions in the regulation of food intake. Proc Nutr Soc. 2007;66(1):131–55.

9. Gao Q, Horvath TL. Neurobiology of feeding and energy expenditure. Annu Rev Neurosci. 2007;30:367–98.
10. Morgan MJ, Liu ZG. Crosstalk of reactive oxygen species and NF-κB signaling. Cell Res. 2011;21(1):103–15.
11. Finkel T. Signal transduction by reactive oxygen species. J Cell Biol. 2011;194(1):7–15.
12. Federico A, Cardaioli E, Da Pozzo P, Formichi P, Gallus GN, Radi E. Mitochondria, oxidative stress and neurodegeneration. J Neurol Sci. 2012;322(1–2):254–62.
13. Zhang X, Dong F, Ren J, Driscoll MJ, Culver B. High dietary fat induces NADPH oxidase-associated oxidative stress and inflammation in rat cerebral cortex. Exp Neurol. 2005;191(2):318–25.
14. Parton LE, Ye CP, Coppari R, et al. Glucose sensing by POMC neurons regulates glucose homeostasis and is impaired in obesity. Nature. 2007;449(7159):228–32.
15. Lin J, Wu PH, Tarr PT, et al. Defects in adaptive energy metabolism with CNS-linked hyperactivity in PGC-1alpha null mice. Cell. 2004;119(1):121–35.
16. Tabas I, Ron D. Integrating the mechanisms of apoptosis induced by endoplasmic reticulum stress. Nat Cell Biol. 2011;13(3):184–90.
17. Hotamisligil GS. Endoplasmic reticulum stress and the inflammatory basis of metabolic disease. Cell. 2010;140(6):900–17.
18. Denis RG, Arruda AP, Romanatto T, et al. TNF-α transiently induces endoplasmic reticulum stress and an incomplete unfolded protein response in the hypothalamus. Neuroscience. 2010;170(4):1035–44.
19. Won JC, Jang PG, Namkoong C, et al. Central administration of an endoplasmic reticulum stress inducer inhibits the anorexigenic effects of leptin and insulin. Obesity. 2009;17(10):1861–5.
20. Zhang X, Zhang G, Zhang H, Karin M, Bai H, Cai D. Hypothalamic IKKbeta/NF-kappaB and ER stress link overnutrition to energy imbalance and obesity. Cell. 2008;135(1):61–73.
21. Levine B, Kroemer G. Autophagy in the pathogenesis of disease. Cell. 2008;132(1):27–42.
22. Klionsky DJ. Autophagy: from phenomenology to molecular understanding in less than a decade. Nat Rev Mol Cell Biol. 2007;8:931–7.
23. Komatsu M, Waguri S, Ueno T, et al. Impairment of starvation-induced and constitutive autophagy in Atg7-deficiente mice. J Cell Biol. 2005;169(3):425–34.
24. Levine B. Eating oneself and uninvited guests: autophagy-related pathways in cellular defense. Cell. 2005;120(2):159–62.
25. Shintani T, Klionsky DJ. Autophagy in health and disease: a double-edged sword. Science. 2004;306(5698):990–5.
26. Yang L, Li P, Fu S, Calay ES, Hotamisligil GS. Defective hepatic autophagy in obesity promotes ER stress and causes insulin resistance. Cell Metab. 2010;11(6):467–78.
27. Masiero E, Agatea L, Mammucari C, et al. Autophagy is required to maintain muscle mass. Cell Metab. 2009;10(6):507–15.
28. Fujitani Y, Kawamori R, Watada H. The role of autophagy in pancreatic beta-cell and diabetes. Autophagy. 2009;5(2):280–2.
29. Martinez-Vicente M, Cuervo AM. Autophagy and neurodegeneration: when the cleaning crew goes on strike. Lancet Neurol. 2007;6(4):352–61.
30. Meng Q, Cai D. Defective hypothalamic autophagy directs the central pathogenesis of obesity via the IkappaB kinase beta (IKKbeta)/NF-kappaB pathway. J Biol Chem. 2011;286(37):32324–32.
31. Schwartz M, Moalem G, Leibowitz-Amit R, Cohen IR. Innate and adaptive immune responses can be beneficial for CNS repair. Trends Neurosci. 1999;22(7):295–9.
32. Fessler MB, Rudel LL, Brown JM. Toll-like receptor signaling links dietary fatty acids to the metabolic syndrome. Curr Opin Lipidol. 2009;20(5):379–85.
33. Milanski M, Degasperi G, Coope A, et al. Saturated fatty acids produce an inflammatory response predominantly through the activation of TLR4 signaling in hypothalamus: implications for the pathogenesis of obesity. J Neurosci. 2009;29(2):359–70.

34. Kleinridders A, Schenten D, Könner AC, et al. MyD88 signaling in the CNS is required for development of fatty acid-induced leptin resistance and diet-induced obesity. Cell Metab. 2009;10(4):249–59.
35. Ferrante Jr AW. Obesity-induced inflammation: a metabolic dialogue in the language of inflammation. J Intern Med. 2007;262(4):408–14.
36. Romanatto T, Cesquini M, Amaral ME, et al. TNF-alpha acts in the hypothalamus inhibiting food intake and increasing the respiratory quotient-effects on leptin and insulin signaling pathways. Peptides. 2007;28(5):1050–8.
37. Uysal KT, Wiesbrock SM, Marino MW, Hotamisligil GS. Protection from obesity-induced insulin resistance in mice lacking TNF-alpha function. Nature. 1997;389(6651):610–4.
38. Ropelle ER, Flores MB, Cintra DE, et al. IL-6 and IL-10 anti-inflammatory activity links exercise to hypothalamic insulin and leptin sensitivity through IKKbeta and ER stress inhibition. PLoS Biol. 2010;8:e1000465.
39. Vaughan S, Jat PS. Deciphering the role of nuclear factor-κB in cellular senescence. Aging (Albany NY). 2011;3(10):913–9.
40. Canty Jr TG, Boyle Jr AE, Farr A, Morgan EN, Verrier ED, Pohlman TH. Oxidative stress induces NF-kappaB nuclear translocation without degradation of IkappaBalpha. Circulation. 1999;100(19 Suppl):II361–4.
41. Herscovitch M, Comb W, Ennis T, et al. Intermolecular disulfide bond formation in the NEMO dimer requires Cys54 and Cys347. Biochem Biophys Res Commun. 2008;367(1):103–8.
42. Christman KW, Blackwell TS, Juurlink BH. Redox regulation of nuclear factor kappa B: therapeutic potential for attenuating inflammatory responses. Brain Pathol. 2000;10(1):153–62.
43. Song YS, Kim MS, Kim HA, et al. Oxidative stress increases phosphorylation of IkappaB kinase-alpha by enhancing NF-kappaB-inducing kinase after transient focal cerebral ischemia. J Cereb Blood Flow Metab. 2010;30(7):1265–74.
44. Lezoualc'h F, Behl C. Transcription factor NF-kappaB: friend or foe of neurons? Mol Psychiatry. 1998;3(1):15–20.
45. Stein S, Schäfer N, Breitenstein A, et al. SIRT1 reduces endothelial activation without affecting vascular function in ApoE–/– mice. Aging (Albany NY). 2010;2(6):353–60.
46. Purkayastha S, Zhang H, Zhang G, Ahmed Z, Wang Y, Cai D. Neural dysregulation of peripheral insulin action and blood pressure by brain endoplasmic reticulum stress. Proc Natl Acad Sci U S A. 2011;108(7):2939–44.
47. Oh-I S, Thaler JP, Ogimoto K, Wisse BE, Morton GJ, Schwartz MW. Central administration of interleukin-4 exacerbates hypothalamic inflammation and weight gain during high-fat feeding. Am J Physiol Endocrinol Metab. 2010;299(1):E47–53.
48. Cai D, Liu T. Inflammatory cause of metabolic syndrome via brain stress and NF-κB. Aging (Albany NY). 2012;4(2):98–115.
49. Li J, Tang Y, Cai D. IKKβ/NF-κB disrupts adult hypothalamic neural stem cells to mediate a neurodegenerative mechanism of dietary obesity and pre-diabetes. Nat Cell Biol. 2012;14(10):999–1012.
50. McNay DE, Briançon N, Kokoeva MV, Maratos-Flier E, Flier JS. Remodeling of the arcuate nucleus energy-balance circuit is inhibited in obese mice. J Clin Invest. 2012;122(1):142–52.
51. Gage FH. Mammalian neural stem cells. Science. 2000;287(5457):1433–8.
52. Gould E. How widespread is adult neurogenesis in mammals? Nat Rev Neurosci. 2007;8(6):481–8.
53. Kokoeva MV, Yin H, Flier JS. Evidence for constitutive neural cell proliferation in the adult murine hypothalamus. J Comp Neurol. 2007;505(2):209–20.
54. Kokoeva MV, Yin H, Flier JS. Neurogenesis in the hypothalamus of adult mice: potential role in energy balance. Science. 2005;310(5748):679–83.

55. Pierce AA, Xu AW. De novo neurogenesis in adult hypothalamus as a compensatory mechanism to regulate energy balance. J Neurosci. 2010;30(2):723–30.
56. Cai D. Neuroinflammation and neurodegeneration in overnutrition-induced diseases. Trends Endocrinol Metab. 2013;24(1):40–7.
57. Posey KA, Clegg DJ, Printz RL, et al. Hypothalamic proinflammatory lipid accumulation, inflammation, and insulin resistance in rats fed a high-fat diet. Am J Physiol Endocrinol Metab. 2009;296(5):E1003–12.
58. Kievit P, Howard JK, Badman MK, et al. Enhanced leptin sensitivity and improved glucose homeostasis in mice lacking suppressor of cytokine signaling-3 in POMC-expressing cells. Cell Metab. 2006;4(2):123–32.
59. Gao Z, Yin J, Zhang J, He Q, McGuinness OP, Ye J. Inactivation of NF-kappaB p50 leads to insulin sensitization on liver through post-translational inhibition of p70S6K. J Biol Chem. 2009;284(27):18368–76.
60. Boaz M, Lisy L, Zandman-Goddard G, Wainstein J. The effect of anti-inflammatory (aspirin and/or statin) therapy on body weight in Type 2 diabetic individuals: EAT, a retrospective study. Diabet Med. 2009;26(7):708–13.
61. Duffy D, Rader D. Endocannabinoid antagonism: blocking the excess in the treatment of high-risk abdominal obesity. Trends Cardiovasc Med. 2007;17(2):35–43.
62. Ozcan U, Yilmaz E, Ozcan L, et al. Chemical chaperones reduce ER stress and restore glucose homeostasis in a mouse model of type 2 diabetes. Science. 2006;313(5790):1137–40.
63. Kars M, Yang L, Gregor MF, et al. Tauroursodeoxycholic Acid may improve liver and muscle but not adipose tissue insulin sensitivity in obese men and women. Diabetes. 2010;59(8):1899–905.
64. Fleischman A, Johnsen S, Systrom DM, et al. Effects of a nucleoside reverse transcriptase inhibitor, stavudine, on glucose disposal and mitochondrial function in muscle of healthy adults. Am J Physiol Endocrinol Metab. 2007;292(6):E1666–73.
65. Weseler AR, Bast A. Oxidative stress and vascular function: implications for pharmacologic treatments. Curr Hypertens Rep. 2010;12(3):154–61.
66. Purkayastha S, Zhang G, Cai D. Uncoupling the mechanisms of obesity and hypertension by targeting hypothalamic IKK-β and NF-κB. Nat Med. 2011;17(7):883–7.
67. Corder EH, Saunders AM, Strittmatter WJ. Gene dose of apolipoprotein E type 4 allele and the risk of Alzheimer's Disease in late-onset families. Science. 1993;261(5123):921–31.
68. Sena A, Capela C, Nóbrega C, Férret-Sena V, Campos E, Pedrosa R. Chapter 23: Plasma lipoproteins in brain inflammatory and neurodegenerative diseases. In: Lipoproteins – role in health and diseases. Frank S, Koster G (Eds). Intech; 2012:564–582.
69. Bell R, Zlokovic B. Neurovascular mechanisms and blood–brain barrier disorder in Alzheimer's disease. Acta Neuropathol. 2009;118(1):103–13.
70. Perry VH, Holmes C. Microglial priming in neurodegenerative disease. Nat Rev Neurol. 2014;10(4):217–24.
71. Holmes C, Cunningham C, Zotova E, Culliford D, Perry VH. Proinflammatory cytokines, sickness behavior, and Alzheimer disease. Neurology. 2011;77(3):212–8.
72. van den Berg E, Biessels GJ, de Craen AJ, Gussekloo J, Westendorp RG. The metabolic syndrome is associated with decelerated cognitive decline in the oldest old. Neurology. 2007;69(10):979–85.
73. Forti P, Pisacane N, Rietti E, Lucicesare A, Olivelli V, Mariani E, et al. Metabolic syndrome and risk of dementia in older adults. J Am Geriatr Soc. 2010;58(3):487–92.
74. Lionetti L, Mollica MP, Lombardi A, Cavaliere G, Gifuni G, Barletta A. From chronic overnutrition to insulin resistance: the role of fat-storing capacity and inflammation. Nutr Metab Cardiovasc Dis. 2009;19(2):146–52.
75. Prieur X, Roszer T, Ricote M. Lipotoxicity in macrophages: evidence from diseases associated with the metabolic syndrome. Biochim Biophys Acta. 2009;1801(3):327–37.
76. Watts A, Loskutova N, Burns J, Johnson D. Metabolic syndrome and cognitive decline in early Alzheimer's disease and healthy older adults. J Alzheimers Dis. 2013;35(2):253–65.

77. Song J, Lee JE. Adiponectin as a new paradigm for approaching Alzheimer's disease. Anat Cell Biol. 2013;46(4):229–34.
78. Bhat N. Linking cardiometabolic disorders to sporadic AD: a perspective on potential mechanisms and mediators. J Neurochem. 2010;115(3):551–62.
79. Kiliaan AJ, Arnoldussen IAC, Gustafson DR. Adipokines: a link between obesity and dementia? Lancet Neurol. 2014;13(9):913–23.
80. Hall J, Wiechmann AR, Johnson LA, Edwards M, Barber RC, Winter AS, et al. Biomarkers of vascular risk, systemic inflammation and microvascular pathology and neuropsychiatric symptoms in Alzheimer's disease. J Alzheimers Dis. 2013;35(2):363–71.
81. Vikarunnessa S, Weiner M, Vega GL. LDL phenotype in subjects with mild cognitive impairment and Alzheimer's disease. J Alzheimers Dis. 2013;36(3):571–5.
82. Engelhart MJ, Geerlings MI, Meijer J, Kiliaan A, Ruitenberg A, van Swieten JC, et al. Inflammatory proteins in plasma and the risk of dementia: the Rotterdam study. Arch Neurol. 2004;61(5):668–72.
83. Tan ZS, Beiser AS, Vasan RS, Roubenoff R, Dinarello CA, Harris TB, et al. Inflammatory markers and the risk of Alzheimer disease: the Framingham Study. Neurology. 2007;68(22):1902–8.
84. Holmes C, Cunningham C, Zotova E, Woolford J, Dean C, Kerr S, et al. Systemic inflammation and disease progression in Alzheimer disease. Neurology. 2009;73(10):768–74.
85. Vlad S, Miller D, Kowall N, Felson D. Protective effects of NSAIDs on the development of Alzheimer disease. Neurology. 2008;70(19):1672–7.
86. McGeer PL, McGeer EG. NSAIDs and Alzheimer disease: epidemiological, animal model and clinical studies. Neurobiol Aging. 2007;28(5):639–47.
87. Grammas P. Neurovascular dysfunction, inflammation and endothelial activation: implications for the pathogenesis of Alzheimer's disease. J Neuroinflammation. 2014;8(1):26.
88. Wong WB, Lin VW, Boudreau D, Devine EB. Statins in the prevention of dementia and Alzheimer's disease: a meta- analysis of observational studies and an assessment of confounding. Pharmacoepidemiol Drug Safety. 2013;22(4):345–58.
89. Malfitano AM, Marasco G, Proto MC, Laezza C, Gazzerro P, Bifulco M. Statins in neurological disorders: an overview and update. Pharmacol Res. 2014;88:74–83.
90. Craft S, Baker LD, Montine TJ, Minoshima S, Watson GS, Claxton A, et al. Intranasal insulin therapy for Alzheimer disease and amnestic mild cognitive impairment: a pilot clinical trial. Arch Neurol. 2012;69(1):29–38.
91. Reger MA, Watson GS, Green PS, Wilkinson CW, Baker LD, Cholerton B, et al. Intranasal insulin improves cognition and modulates beta-amyloid in early AD. Neurology. 2008;70(6):440–8.
92. Cheng X, Shen Y, Li R. Targeting TNF: a therapeutic strategy for Alzheimer's disease. Drug Discov Today. 2014;4:1–6.
93. Martins IJ, Hone E, Foster JK, Sünram-Lea SI, Gnjec A, Fuller SJ, et al. Apolipoprotein E, cholesterol metabolism, diabetes, and the convergence of risk factors for Alzheimer's disease and cardiovascular disease. Mol Psychiatry. 2006;11(8):721–36.
94. Gu Y, Luchsinger JA, Stern Y, Scarmeas N. Mediterranean diet, inflammatory and metabolic biomarkers, and risk of Alzheimer's disease. J Alzheimers Dis. 2010;22(2):483–92.
95. Braskie MN, Boyle CP, Rajagopalan P, Gutman BA, Toga AW, Raji CA, et al. Physical activity, inflammation, and volume of the aging brain. Neuroscience. 2014;273:199–209.
96. Duarte JM, Schuck PF, Wenk GL, Ferreira GC. Metabolic disturbances in diseases with neurological involvement. Aging Dis. 2014;5(4):238–55.
97. Friese MA, Schattling B, Fugger L. Mechanisms of neurodegeneration and axonal dysfunction in multiple sclerosis. Nat Rev Neuro. 2014;10(4):225–38.
98. Ramagopalan SV, Dobson R, Meier UC, Giovannoni G. Multiple sclerosis: risk factors, prodromes, and potential causal pathways. Lancet Neurol. 2010;9(7):727–39.

99. Martins TB, Rose JW, Jaskowski TD, Wilson AR, Husebye D, Seraj HS, et al. Analysis of proinflammatory and anti-inflammatory cytokine serum concentrations in patients with multiple sclerosis by using a multiplexed immunoassay. Am J Clin Pathol. 2011;136(5):696–704.
100. Hernández-Pedro NY, Espinosa-Ramirez G, de la Cruz VP, Pineda B, Sotelo J. Initial immunopathogenesis of multiple sclerosis: innate immune response. Clin Dev Immunol. 2013;2013:413465.
101. Correale J. The role of microglial activation in disease progression. Mult Scler. 2014;20(10):1288–95.
102. Moreno B, Jukes J-P, Vergara-Irigaray N, Errea O, Villoslada P, Perry VH, et al. Systemic inflammation induces axon injury during brain inflammation. Ann Neurol. 2011;70(6):932–42.
103. Wens I, Dalgas U, Stenager E, Eijnde BO. Risk factors related to cardiovascular diseases and the metabolic syndrome in multiple sclerosis - a systematic review. Mult Scler. 2013;19(12):1556–64.
104. LaVela SL, Prohaska TR, Furner S, Weaver FM. Chronic diseases in male veterans with multiple sclerosis. Prev Chronic Dis. 2012;9(3):E55.
105. Christiansen CF. Risk of vascular disease in patients with multiple sclerosis: a review. Neurol Res. 2012;34(8):746–53.
106. Jadidi E, Mohammadi M, Moradi T. High risk of vascular diseases after diagnosis of multiple sclerosis. Mult Scler. 2013;19(10):1336–40.
107. Marrie RA, Rudick R, Horwitz R, Cutter G, Tyry T, Campagnolo D, et al. Vascular comorbidity is associated with more rapid disability progression in multiple sclerosis. Neurology. 2010;74(13):1041–7.
108. Palavra F, Marado D, Mascarenhas-Melo F, Sereno J, Teixeira-Lemos E, Nunes CC, et al. New markers of early cardiovascular risk in multiple sclerosis patients: oxidized-LDL correlates with clinical staging. Dis Markers. 2013;34(5):341–8.
109. Tettey P, Simpson S, Taylor B, Blizzard L, Ponsonby AL, Dwyer T, et al. An adverse lipid profile is associated with disability and progression of disability, in people with MS. Mult Scler. 2014;20(13):1737–44.
110. Weinstock-Guttman B, Zivadinov R, Mahfooz N, Carl E, Drake A, Schneider J, et al. Serum lipid profiles are associated with disability and MRI outcomes in multiple sclerosis. J Neuroinflammation. 2011;8:127.
111. Ciurleo R, Bramanti P, Marino S. Role of statins in the treatment of multiple sclerosis. Pharmacol Res. 2014;87:133–43.
112. Chataway J, Schuerer N, Alsanousi A, Chand D, MacManus D, Hunter K, et al. Effect of high-dose simvastatin on brain atrophy and disability in secondary progressive multiple sclerosis (MS-STAT): a randomised, placebo-controlled, phase 2 trial. Lancet. 2014;383(9936):2213–21.
113. Feng X, Han D, Kilaru B, Franek BS, Niewold TB, Reder AT. Inhibition of interferon-beta responses in multiple sclerosis immune cells associated with high-dose statins. Arch Neurol. 2012;69(10):1303–9..
114. Sena A, Pedrosa R, Morais MG. Beneficial effect of statins in multiple sclerosis: is it dose-dependent? Atherosclerosis. 2007;191(2):462.
115. Sena A, Pedrosa R, Morais MG. Statins for multiple sclerosis. Lancet. 2004;364(9432):412.
116. Sena A, Pedrosa R, Graça MM. Therapeutic potential of lovastatin in multiple sclerosis. J Neurol. 2003;250(6):754–5.
117. Matarese G, Procaccini C, De Rosa V. The intricate interface between immune and metabolic regulation: a role for leptin in the pathogenesis of multiple sclerosis? J Leukoc Biol. 2008;84(4):893–9.
118. Munger KL, Chitnis T, Ascherio A. Body size and risk of MS in two cohorts of US women. Neurology. 2009;73(19):1543–50.
119. Hedström AK, Lima Bomfim I, Barcellos L, Gianfrancesco M, Schaefer C, Kockum I, et al. Interaction between adolescent obesity and HLA risk genes in the etiology of multiple sclerosis. Neurology. 2014;82(10):865–72.

120. Wöbke TK, Sorg BL, Steinhilber D. Vitamin D in inflammatory diseases. Front Physiol. 2014;5:244.
121. Oliveira SR, Simão AN, Kallaur AP, de Almeida ER, Morimoto HK, Lopes J, et al. Disability in patients with multiple sclerosis: influence of insulin resistance, adiposity, and oxidative stress. Nutrition. 2014;30(3):268–73.
122. Farez MF, Fiol MP, Gaitán MI, Quintana FJ, Correale J. Sodium intake is associated with increased disease activity in multiple sclerosis. J Neurol Neurosurg Psychiatry. 2015;86(1):26–31.
123. Collins LM, Toulouse A, Connor TJ, Nolan YM. Contributions of central and systemic inflammation to the pathophysiology of Parkinson's disease. Neuropharmacology. 2012;62(7):2154–68.
124. Maes M. An intriguing and hitherto unexplained co-occurrence: depression and chronic fatigue syndrome are manifestations of shared inflammatory, oxidative and nitrosative (IO&NS) pathways. Prog Neuropsychopharmacol Biol Pshychiatry. 2011;35(3):784–94.
125. Cunningham C. Microglia and neurodegeneration: the role of systemic inflammation. Glia. 2013;61(1):71–90.

Index

© Springer International Publishing Switzerland 2015
F. Palavra et al. (eds.), *Biomarkers of Cardiometabolic Risk, Inflammation and Disease*, DOI 10.1007/978-3-319-16018-4

MIX
Papier aus verantwortungsvollen Quellen
Paper from responsible sources
FSC® C105338

If you have any concerns about our products,
you can contact us on
ProductSafety@springernature.com

In case Publisher is established outside the EU,
the EU authorized representative is:
Springer Nature Customer Service Center GmbH
Europaplatz 3, 69115 Heidelberg, Germany

Printed by Libri Plureos GmbH
in Hamburg, Germany